Metamorphoses of Psyche in Psychoanalysis and Ancient Greek Thought

This unusual book explores the transformative power of liminal experiences in ancient Greek texts, psychoanalytic theory, and the author's own life, to demonstrate how a contemporary understanding of ancient thought can illuminate modern psychoanalytic theory and practice especially as it relates to trauma, grief, and the development of psyche.

With the understanding that liminal experiencing involves engaging a psychic space outside the boundaries of ego organization, Dobson artfully interweaves autobiography, literary analysis, philosophical ontology, and psychoanalysis, to formulate a new paradigm for how to construct human beings, how to enliven and deepen personal and therapeutic experience, and how poetic language is a gateway to this magical realm of transformation. Alongside richly detailed case analyses, the author uses her dual expertise in psychoanalysis and ancient Greek literature to explore how the maternal and liminal in human life were displaced with the rise of Athens and a new way of being human – the rational citizen – and how this repression has resulted in diminished, constricted experiencing and the suppression of women throughout western history.

With a deep understanding of classical literature and psychoanalysis, and extensive clinical insights, this is essential reading for psychoanalysts, psychotherapists, classicists, and historians wishing to understand how ancient thought and modern psychoanalysis can interact.

Marcia D-S. Dobson has PhDs in Classical Philology and Clinical Psychology. She has been an award-winning Professor of Classics at Colorado College for over 40 years and has a private psychotherapy practice in Colorado Springs, Colorado.

Art, Creativity, and Psychoanalysis Book Series
George Hagman, LCSW

Series Editor

The *Art, Creativity, and Psychoanalysis* book series seeks to highlight original, cutting-edge studies of the relationship between psychoanalysis and the world of art and the psychology of artists, with subject matter including the psychobiography of artists, the creative process, the psychology of aesthetic experience, as well as the aesthetic, creative, and artistic aspects of psychoanalysis and psychoanalytic psychotherapy. *Art, Creativity, and Psychoanalysis* promotes a vision of psychoanalysis as a creative art, the clinical effectiveness of which can be enhanced when we better understand and utilize artistic and creative processes at its core.

The series welcomes proposals from psychoanalytic therapists from all professional groups and theoretical models, as well as artists, art historians, and art critics informed by a psychoanalytic perspective. For a full list of all titles in the series, please visit the Routledge website at: https://www.routledge.com/ACAPBS.

Poetry and Psychoanalysis
The Opening of the Field
David Shaddock

Affect in Artistic Creativity
Painting to Feel
Jussi Saarinen

Scansion in Psychoanalysis and Art
The Cut in Creation
Vanessa Sinclair

Metamorphoses of Psyche in Psychoanalysis and Ancient Greek Thought

From Mourning to Creativity

Marcia D-S. Dobson

Routledge
Taylor & Francis Group
LONDON AND NEW YORK

Cover image: "Pele Dreaming", Copyright Herbert K. Kane, LLX

First published 2023
by Routledge
4 Park Square, Milton Park, Abingdon, Oxon OX14 4RN

and by Routledge
605 Third Avenue, New York, NY 10158

Routledge is an imprint of the Taylor & Francis Group, an informa business

British Library Cataloguing-in-Publication Data
A catalogue record for this book is available from the British Library

ISBN: 9781032375519 (hbk)
ISBN: 9781032375526 (pbk)
ISBN: 9781003340751 (ebk)

DOI: 10.4324/9781003340751

Typeset in Times New Roman
by Newgen Publishing UK

To my parents,
Helen Flanders Dunbar, MD,
and George Henry Soule, Jr.
In memoriam
*
To my husband, John Hanwell Riker,
and my daughter, Sophia Flanders Mendoza.
With endless love for all you are and all the good you do

Contents

Preface by Series Editor

George Hagman

This wonderful book, *Metamorphoses of Psyche in Psychoanalysis and Ancient Greek Thought: From Mourning to Creativity* by Marcia Dobson, is the sixth volume in the book series Art, Creativity, and Psychoanalysis published by Routledge. In it, Dobson takes the reader on a journey in the deepest, most passionate and risky sense, through the psychological and cultural space between personal experience, art and psychoanalysis within which beauty and truth reside. This book is full to the brim with knowledge, sadness, love and longing as well as a generous, healing sensibility. Most important, it is a self-portrait of a scholar, artist, and therapist who finds both great tragedy and joy in life.

It is the type of book that I was hoping for when we initiated the Art, Creativity and Psychoanalysis (ACP) book series. Traditionally, art and creativity have been areas for "applied psychoanalysis," an extra, albeit fascinating area of human experience, which psychoanalysis, in addition to its primary clinical purpose, can help to illuminate. However, for the authors in the ACP series, art and psychoanalysis are one; they believe that beauty and creativity are at the heart of human experience and clinical practice. We long for beauty as we long for sex. The capacity to live creatively is the very definition of mental health. We are all "artists of our lives" as Adam Phillips writes.

Dobson knows this in her bones. As you read her book, you feel that she actually lived among the ancient Greeks, reading editions of Homer, Aeschylus, Sophocles, Euripides, and Ovid in their original languages of Greek and Latin, and attending the performances of ancient Greek tragedy, such as Sophocles' Oedipus, or Euripides' "Medea," which would come to so profoundly influence the sensibility of Freud and the body of psychoanalytic thought. She can describe how those ancient texts are still vitally relevant to us, and how the profound truths that they describe are still relevant to modern life and psychoanalytic practice.

But even more important, with honesty and great compassion she shares her own history of loss, trauma, and recovery to demonstrate how the arts and aesthetics can capture the most tragic of human experiences, and the core of pain and loss which plague us. Yet she also asserts from personal experience the healing power of psychoanalysis and the psychoanalytic relationship, and how all of it, art, tragedy, and analysis, can come together within a single person's sense of self.

It is how we live our lives which preoccupies Dobson. For most of us, our days are dominated and constrained by fact, explanation, and a need to know the answer. Dobson encourages us to cultivate a liminal attitude, or more precisely a liminal state of mind, in which we are poised at the threshold of being, allowing the mysterious and unpredictable to enter our lives, when we encounter the unexpected, strange, and wonderful. In this sense, psychoanalysis and art are aspects of "creative living" as Winnicott described, in which vital and healthy selfhood is always open to experience, resourceful and hopefully wise. If we are lucky, it is in this receptiveness and ever renewing creative capacity that truth and beauty can be found; and in this way, as in Dobson's book, scholarship, writing, and therapy can be acts of creativity and love.

Author's Preface

Poetry, painting, sculpture, and the many other arts hold us and teach us who we are. These are aesthetic languages in which the psyche expresses itself with both sense and feeling. The space in which these aesthetic realms come into being is liminal and transformational. This is how they open us to a world that is ever changing, while giving us the possibility to feel at home in that change. In my own life these languages were born and flourished through grieving.

Psychoanalysis in its many relational and intersubjective forms creates itself through liminal sensibilities – that is, by dwelling in spaces between, around, and within patient and therapist so as to bring about healing and transformation for them both. For me it is most affective and effective when it thinks in aesthetic language.

Indeed, psychoanalysis is itself an art, and we are artists. But how is it that we are artists? And what is it that so deeply connects us to aesthetic language and the third spaces it dwells in – liminal spaces – where the creativity lying deep within the known and yet unknown in us can lead to transformative ways of being? This book intermingles autobiography, psychoanalytic theory, and ancient Greek literature in the hopes of being one kind of answer to that question.

I am influenced throughout by my personal and professional life story. I am writing intentionally in a personal and subjective voice, exploring my own life experiences with dreams, myths, spirituality, ancient Greek literature, and clinical work, as a scholar, a patient, and a therapist. I confess that in my attempts to make psychoanalysis more accessible to classicists as a way to understand the ancient Greeks I have left out some of the specificities of theory and practice to which psychotherapists and psychoanalysts are accustomed. I have also left out many of the demands for the philological precision that classicists insist on in their own research in my desire to welcome them into the new languages of psychoanalysis as a tool for their own interpretations of the ancient Greeks. I hope that my intertwining of these two fields creates not only new ways to think about both psychoanalysis and ancient Greek literature, but also generates a new vision for how to construct human experience.

I do not expect that my own idiosyncratic personal journey will be anything like those of others, but I am retelling it in the hopes that it will help both clinicians and classicists to become more open and empathic to their own experiences with liminal realms and consider how such experiences can lead to interconnectedness with others.

Over the years of writing this book, I have become aware that a growing number of my colleagues are also sensing and expressing the magnitude of a paradigm shift in the way we are living in the world. Something mysteriously beyond us seems, indeed, to be calling to us to express new meanings about how to live empathically in and with diversity, otherness, and the whole.

At the most recent International Association for Psychoanalytic Self Psychology Conference, I rejoiced hearing Raanan Kulka's introductory words:

> The feasibility of a spiritual psychoanalytic thinking originated in the conceptual passage from the Guilty man and the Tragic man to the Mystic man, and it springs from a shift from a psychoanalysis based on an orientation of separateness towards a psychoanalysis anchored in a unified world-view of Oneness."
>
> ("The Spiritual Core of Kohut's Legacy."
> January 26, 2022)

Across the seas, oceans, mountains, and blue sky of the Mediterranean from Israel to Colorado, my own home, the infinitely Hermes-like swiftness of our modern internet spins me into a liminal space of recognition of how the human being at once "emerges into individual existence, and dissolves into the transcendent being of supra-individual existence of participation in the world" (Kulka, 2021).

I do not write alone.

Reference

Kulka, R. (2021). Self psychology: The ethics of oneness. *Psychoanalytic Review* 108: 141–153.

Acknowledgments

This book could not have come into existence without the help of many people whom I would like to acknowledge. Dr. Jeffrey Stern and Suzi Naiburg are the close editors to whom I owe the debt of writing in a less "oracular" style that has, I hope, turned out in the end to be an English that my readers might understand and even, at moments, enjoy reading. Dr. Bennett Simon, author of *Mind and Madness in Ancient Greece*, has helped immeasurably in conversing with me about the views I have put forward on the ancient Greeks, and our delightful conversations have prepared me for inevitable but stimulating collegial battles. Both he and Dr. Peter Rudnytsky, who has read the full text, are scholars of the Greeks and psychoanalysis, and know perhaps better than anyone the vicissitudes of working in two fields simultaneously. Dr. Kathryn Kuisle, a diplomate Jungian analyst, has followed this book chapter by chapter, reassuring me in my efforts to bridge Jungian and psychoanalytic understandings, and telling me, as have many others, that it is alright to be personal in my literary style.

I owe a deep debt of gratitude to my "writing sisters" Drs. Brenda Solomon, Karen Martin, and Carol Mayhew, who have been guides and enthusiasts throughout our creative, clinical writing journeys with Suzi Naiburg over our years together. I want to thank as well the students who have taken the time and effort to comment on my chapters and to give me invaluable feedback, not to mention all my own teachers through the years from both Pacifica Graduate Institute and Harvard University, who have taught me so much of what I know.

I am especially beholden to Dr. Raanan Kulka, who has turned out to be a soulmate across the miles and who shares my beliefs about spirituality and oneness. It is remarkable to find such a rare friend.

Above all, my husband John H. Riker, a philosopher of the psychology of Kohut and my partner in a life of writing, teaching, loving, and ballroom dancing, has read every word of this manuscript more than once, and has held my hand throughout my sudden descents into the impossibilities of saying what I need to say, encouraging me always to speak from the honesty of my convictions, even in my darkest hours about the possibility of doing so.

I am also deeply grateful to Professor Sanjaya Thakur, the Chair of Classics at Colorado College, who has opened my eyes to the brilliance of Ovid, respected my deep commitment to writing this book, and given me the time to do so, and to our administrative assistant, Eileen Broderick, who helped prepare the manuscript.

Last and first, I owe the deepest thanks to my patients, without whom I could never have written this book. Through you I have found, and keep finding out, who I am and who we are. You have become a part of me.

Dr. George Hagman, the Editor of this series on Art, Psychoanalysis and Creativity, accepted the proposal for the book, and without him it might never have been published. Thank you, George, for your own writing, which has helped me and so many of my students to understand and move through grieving, and for your own extraordinary journey from the subject of mourning to that of creativity, which so closely mirrors my own.

Part I

A Search for the Self Through Liminal Experiences

Chapter 1

Introduction

1.1 The Nature of Liminal and Imaginal Experiences

It is October, 1998. I am a fledgling therapist sitting in a rented office on the first floor of a pale blue turn-of-the-century Victorian building. Across from me is a windowed wall with a flowered couch in front of it on which my new patient is sitting. There is a coffee table positioned between us, and a small, now dying, kitchen garden outside the windows. The sun is setting, casting long shadows across the room. A grandfather clock stands against the wall to my right, and an old rocking chair. Both are just out of my eyesight.

My patient and I are caught in silence. The sound of the tall clock ticking grows louder. And then, inexplicably, the chair begins to creak, as if someone is sitting in it. I feel I mustn't take my eyes from my patient, but I am startled, curious, and a little shaken. I steal a glance. In the chair is the ghostly figure of an old woman, rocking. I try to maintain my composure and turn back to look at my patient. Her face settles into what I imagine to be a deep and painful sadness. Another short silence passes, and then she says: "It's all about my grandmother."

I recall a phrase that I once heard: "When there is an unexpected silence, it means that Hermes has entered the room." Hermes, Greek god of boundaries and crossroads, divine traveler with winged feet and a caduceus, who can bring the dead to life, speed them to Olympus, or give them healing plants to

DOI: 10.4324/9781003340751-2

put them to sleep or transform their minds. I remember, too, the words a psychoanalyst once quoted to me about what another psychoanalyst said: "When there is silence in the room, God is there." In the long shadows of the room that early evening long ago, words and images arise as my patient stutters into truths too unbearable to tell.

In these kinds of liminal or threshold spaces synchronicities stop me suddenly in amazement at their presence. I find a letter in the mailbox from a long-gone and beloved acquaintance who has been on my mind for weeks. Days later she appears unexpectedly at my front door. I dress in clothes of the same colors that the patient I am thinking most about that day is wearing. It happens again and again. It is here that I find the deepest truth of the intimate relatedness of one human being with another. It is a permeable, flickering realm where intuitions and emotions swell to the surface beyond expectable realities, where I find myself in luminous fields of immediacy that dissolve past, present, future … and human boundaries. Here I am humbled and, just for a moment, I feel at home.

Such moments unnerve me in spite of the momentary, shimmering thrill of seeing beyond the veils of what I understand to be "reality." I wonder who the "I" is that came to be so open to them. My therapeutic training did not include any explanations of such experiences except perhaps as manifestations of psychopathology. I had, of course, heard of visionaries, mystics, and shamans, but they rested safely between the leather covers of antiquated books. I also recall ghost stories told by my equally antiquated forebears.

I have come to believe over the years that my passion for studying liminal landscapes arises from the crowds of shifting images, fantasies, and strangely exotic experiences that constituted my childhood world. Thinking and feeling these realms to be real sustained me and helped me to stay alive. They were essential. Fantasy hideaways became so much a part of my own psychic makeup that, as I look back, I wonder if I wasn't somewhat in danger of slipping out of reality altogether. But ultimately it was this very way of being that led to my ability to become deeply grounded as a self while remaining permeable to an environment that opens easily to nature, community, and the sacred, as well as to other human beings. We are all a part of something much larger that speaks through us. We are here to lend it words and eyes, to be the instruments of its expression.

Liminal experiences are everywhere. Children, young and old, find them in playing and imagining, in myths, fairytales, and heroic narratives. Dancers find them in moments of stillness as they leap and hover in the air, or in the swirling concentric circles of the waltz. Such experiences reside in the intermediacies of our lives, the in-between of things. We feel them in a certain thickening of air when we fall in love, or when we find ourselves in deep, empathic attunement with another in our consulting rooms. In psychology, we speak of liminal, imaginal realms as transitional or transformational spaces that occur when the infant emerges from the matrix of its mother into its own self-perception. Jungians sense archetypal emanations arising from the collective unconscious in their dreams. The relational analyst feels the presence of the analytic third, the deep meditative submergence into the soul of a patient, herself perhaps unable to find words for its expression.

It is liminal spaces that allow the soul itself to emerge into the various languages of art.

In painting, they appear as the creative and dense visual metaphors that arise as artists put brush to canvas or chisels to sculpture; in poetry, images seek to be born through the heart, mind, and blood of the poet. In early Greek philosophy, we recognize how paradoxes throw us into a liminal space that brings body to that which seems beyond language. We see it in the philosophical fragments of Heraclitus, the riddles of oracular language, and the grand metaphors of Aeschylean choruses. These kinds of images feel embodied. Because of the force of their energy, they can transform the human psyche itself as it finds ever new and creative ways to live in our complex worlds.

But how are we to conceptualize this liminal world? What kinds of words will open the door to a different way of being human in the world, a way in which both our psyches and our realities radically transform, a way in which grandmothers long gone can suddenly reappear?

Heraclitus, one of our most famous pre-Socratic philosophers, known as the Riddler, says: "you could not discover the limits of the soul, even if you traveled by every path in order to do so. Such is the depth of its meaning (*logos*)" (fragment 45, tr. Wheelwright, 1996, p. 72). He also says "Although the *logos* is eternally valid, yet men are unable to understand it, both before they have heard it, and even after they have heard it for the first time" (fragment 1, p. 69).

The word *logos* in Greek may best be expressed here with the English word, "meaning," but its most literal translation from the Greek is simply "word." But why is "word" as a translation of *logos* insufficient? And why do we translate "word" as "meaning"?

The first phrase of Heraclitus' fragment – that we don't understand the *logos* even before we have heard it for the first time – brings our minds up short. It seems obvious. The second, "even after we have heard it for the first time," throws us into the form of an actual riddle: "what is it we don't understand both before and after we have heard it for the first time?" The answer is "meaning," or "*logos*" itself. Whether we are talking philosophy or dream, Heraclitus' words throw us into a psychic conundrum that demands our interpretation but for which there is none. It throws us into a mystery whose answer is always just beyond our reach. We think we have grasped it, but like pinning fluttering butterflies on cardboard, we kill the essence of what we seek as we do it. Like a Zen koan, the fragment's ephemeral, riddle-like nature leaves us with a sense of feeling curious, alive, and desirous of spaces that seem apprehensible, but are not.

Despite the evanescent quality of these words, our very lack of ability to grasp what they mean thickens into form. Like a metaphor with many resonances or the condensation of images in a dream, the very absence of the presence of an answer seems to gain substance. Riddles and paradoxes, like poetry, disrupt the rational structures of our egos and present possibilities for opening doors to experiential spaces beyond them that, even though dark and unconscious, feel "tangible." They live in liminal space.

Half a millennium after Heraclitus, in Ephesus, on the shores of the Aegean Sea in Asia Minor, St John the Apostle delivers his Gospel (in Biblical Greek) on the nature of the *logos*. Ephesus was Heraclitus' hometown. It is hard to believe John was not cognizant of what Heraclitus said.

John carries the definition of *logos* further. He begins in a highly poetic style: "In the beginning was the word (*logos)*, and the word (*logos*) was with God, and God was the word (*logos*)" ... A bit further in the text, John calls the *logos* the "true light" that the darkness could not receive. And then, quite startlingly, John adds that the *logos* "became flesh and dwelt among us."

What John has done here is to embody Heraclitus' idea of the ineffability of the *logos*. He explains it as something that human beings can touch, something like ourselves. In saying that the "logos" becomes "flesh," the substance we are made of, *logos* becomes recognizable and relatable. But in saying that this *logos* is made of light, water, and spirit, John describes a different kind of substance within us that we tend not to recognize and that is mysterious.

The condensation and thickness of the *logos* of which John speaks is identified and described in multiple ways in many religions. Sufis call it subtle matter. Mystics in many faiths describe visions not quite as flesh, but formed in an ethereal space. The little Greek Eros is a visible demi-god flying back and forth between Olympus and earth to connect human beings through passionate love.

John's story of word becoming flesh reaches a further sense of the liminal than does Heraclitus. He expresses powerfully the presence of an image that appears to him as substance because it is full of eros, of light, of energy. John's story reveals the nature of human beings as in ourselves occupying liminal space, hovering between two worlds. We use images that through their light and energy create psychic transformations, and awaken our minds to spirit, vitality, and a sense of the sacred.

This book expresses my own experiences of liminal dwelling in three different ways. It follows these experiences from childhood, through my engagement with ancient Greek culture and into my life as a therapist attempting to effect transformations in my patients.

Chapters 2 through 4 articulate how I lived in and through liminal spaces as a child. Most children, especially only, lonely, children, dramatize and live through their imaginations. But looking back, I realize that I wove the inconsistent and strangely traumatic realities of my actual days into this softer world of my imaginative play, as if I were its author. This gave me both a sense of safety and somewhat misty perceptions of an apparently more substantial actuality. In attempting to make sense of these experiences, I interweave the psychoanalytic theories that most help me to understand them.

These childhood perceptions, as I think upon them today, bear some resemblance to the hauntingly vivid memory of my early patient's grandmother in a rocking chair. In that moment, I perceived in visible form a subject that was shortly to emerge from my patient's own unconscious depths. The unexpressed sorrows she wished to tell me emerged as a visible ghostly but substantial perception prior to her expressing them. Who is to say how her grandmother manifested? My guess is that some riveting relational connection between the two of us brought her into being. The experience of finding my attention drawn to a beloved but long-gone acquaintance who, soon after, unexpectedly appeared in person, or wearing clothes of the same colors as the patient I was most thinking about on her appointment day, engaged me in a similarly unknowable relational field. They all express an experience of connection that is prescient, but not actually present, neither completely invisible, nor fully visible.

In Chapter 3, I further explore what kind of third realm this might be by turning to psychoanalytic developmental theories of liminal and transitional space to interpret early dream experiences, which, once again, have a substantial texture that seemed more real than my waking life. In Chapter 4, I work with my sense of experience of the world, opening beyond my ego boundaries into nature, the sacred, and archetypal mythical realms. In Chapter 5, I describe how the total fragmentation caused by my mother's sudden death by drowning led eventually to profound relational healing and an emerging sense of an expanded, transpersonal self, still focused in liminal dwelling.

Part II of this book opens up an area perhaps less well known to clinicians, that of archaic Greek culture from about 1200–600 BCE. It was this world that I was introduced to early in my life by reading Homer's *Odyssey* in the 6th grade. I read this at the same time that I was reading wonderful children's fairytales and adventure stories, which I quickly adopted as fantasy worlds of my own.

But there was something quite different about the *Odyssey* and Odysseus' adventures. Here I found multiple gods, all of whom seemed to be reverberations of the ancient Greek tribal peoples. It was as if the emotional intensity of their lives was reflected outwards into nature, the sacred, and the community; their emotional and psychic structure did not reside inside of them, but shone throughout the atmosphere for all to see. This world of divinities, as I was later to find out, emerged from an earlier agricultural culture connected with an earth religion based in seasonal cycles of birth, death, and rebirth. Of all the other religions in the Mediterranean, the Greeks shed their animal attributes very early, and grew to stand alone as individuals who were reflected in the gods they created. But even so, their relationship with their gods was vibrant, full of vitality, and resonated with sacred energy.

In Chapter 6, I describe the body of the Greek hero as fluid and unintegrated, more connected to external forces than to itself. In Chapter 7, I show this bodily conception as dwelling in connectivity with the nature and the sacred in such a way that it cannot yet form a coherent model for the western contemporary self. In the Trojan War, the Homeric hero is in disruption, and the male violence in the war seems to be due to a loss of belief in the immortality gained through the agricultural, seasonal cycles of a matricentric world. This necessitates a desperate struggle to gain and hold on to patrilineality, as women and a peaceful agricultural life withdraw further and further afield only to yield a horrifying understanding of individual mortality that can only be assuaged through the lasting glory of the heroic narrative.

In Chapter 8, I work with the rise of the city-state in Aeschylus, and trace a colossal language change as the Homeric hero strides onto the ancient Greek tragic stage and shows his immediate, crippling incapacity to exist in his former heroic glorification in the city-state that is being created.

There has been a paradigm shift. The thick metaphors of Aeschylus in the first play of the *Oresteia*, the "Agamemnon," show us gods distancing themselves and being available only through omen, sign, and oracle – and untrustworthy prophets. Rituals and sacrifices that used to generate the sacred cycling of the seasons are seen as being corrupted by women who formerly were their divine officiants. In the last play, Aeschylus' "Eumenides," former ritual languages of blessing, curse, and magic turn into court language and the rhetoric befitting a city-state. Women themselves are repressed, exiled to the central hearth and the outskirts of the city, but not participating in the city's political life. Finally, Orestes, Clytemnestra's son, commits matricide, only to be purified by Apollo and acquitted in the Areopagus, the Athenian murder court.

Chapter 9 shows the disastrous consequences that occur from the repression of women by taking a look at a few tragedies of Sophocles and the later Euripides, who spotlight heroes, now become brittle, tyrannical, and incapable of ruling precisely because of the loss of the ritual community and the emotional interconnectedness that women can offer. This chapter then returns to the "Homeric Hymn to Demeter" (partially composed in the 8th century BCE), in order to reimagine the ritual world existing before the city-state was created. It suggests that an integration of masculine and feminine values can serve as a model for a stronger, more interconnected psyche essential for our modern western world. Although the internalized psyche of 5th-century Athens with its necessary development of will and self-consciousness has been essential for the development of the western ego, the fear and repression of the feminine has become the Achilles' heel, so to speak, of western culture.

The last and most meditative part of this book evokes my own experiences as a therapist with a theoretical background in psychoanalysis (including Jungian studies, self psychology, and contemporary intersubjective and relational theory). Here, I describe my engagement with two patients through liminal fields that I now accept as a comfortable way of being in the world and a path for finding profound relational interconnectedness. This sense of interconnectedness for me extends not only to others of our own species, but also to natural and metaphysical worlds sensed beyond our conscious awareness. Such fields, evidenced by quantum physics, chaos theory, and other sciences, resonate with depth psychology, mythology, and the aesthetic inspirations of the creative arts.

I am intertwining the three areas of autobiography, archaic Greek literature, and intersubjective, permeable psychodynamic space because each of them reveals something essential about the nature of the liminal. Weaving them together will, I hope, provide a way of grasping this way of perceiving in a complexity and depth not available with only a singular approach. Taken together, they present the possibility for imagining a crucial new construction of the human psyche that can stand as grounds for living a robustly alive and connected human life.

So far, I have spoken of the liminal as it is experienced in philosophical conundrums, in the arts, and in prescient knowing. But we also experience such realms in our readings of fairy tales, myths, and legends, which are like riddles and oracles but take place in the extended time of the narrative form. These narratives open us to imaginal, liminal experiences through stories of heroic journeys of the human psyche. They create parabolic frames for us to find ourselves in. Heroes suffer great adventures in strange, fantastic lands. By traveling on the very edges of the unknown, that is, by exploring liminal spaces, they discover deeper opportunities for the development of their own identities. But such journeys are often fraught with danger and disappointment. These are the liminal paths experienced through time that we meet in third fields in psychotherapy. We take on the figures in our patients' worlds. We are the shapeshifters, inevitably mingling our own stories with theirs even as we accompany and try to guide them on their own journeys.

Our patients suffer what we might call the heroism of mortality. The paths they take with us are of longing and loss, often lying beneath their sense of scintillating grandeur. They, like us, long for perfection and immortality. Stories of such heroes suggest the hope of overcoming the boundaries of human limitations and death and then to return as conquerors, but they are never able to retrieve what they seek. Gilgamesh, the great Mesopotamian hero, journeys to the netherworld to discover the secret to immortality because he so grieves the death of his bosom friend, Enkidu. He is given the challenge not to fall asleep for seven days, but he fails. He plucks the plant that holds the secret to immortality, but it is stolen in the night by a serpent. Orpheus is told he may bring his recently dead wife, Eurydice, back again into the living world, if only he doesn't turn to look at her while in Hades, but he can't resist. These stories suggest that we are willing to chance even death for relationships that can make us feel whole and passionately interconnected. They beckon us to profoundly emotional homes.

But mortal heroes cannot find out who they are without courageous and passionate journeys, which necessitate meeting and connecting with others who are foreign and strange. In doing so, they may discover awful truths about who they are that may destroy them. When Oedipus travels to the Delphic Oracle, the question he asks is "Who am I?" Her response is: "You will kill your father and marry your mother." The answer itself beckons a completely illicit and unspeakable future in riddling form. In short, the question "Who am I?" comes with great dangers of our losing ourselves in chaotic fragmentation, autoeroticism, or narcissistic grandiosity. Such answers are perhaps part of the reason we fear imaginal, liminal experiences and choose to armor ourselves against them.

Many analysts and patients take these dangerous journeys together. It is difficult to encounter such experiences without empathic others beside us to help us to greet the strangers lurking in the wings of our own psyches who seem to be dangerous but hold insights for us. We never quite know the path that is predetermined for us as selves or how we shall ever survive if we really do discover our destinies. But trying to do so is a necessity, because that is how we find our "meaning," even if we can sense it only as mystery.

Human beings have always felt themselves to be at risk in this world precisely because we sense such ambiguities. We live in spaces of unknowing, wishing to know everything. Many of us invest our prophets with holy power because of this. We worship and idealize them. We live in the longing to discover the final truth and the crushing disappointment of its inevitable impossibility. Ancient Greek myth confirms that we are tragic creatures because we long for a truth we can never find fully without being destroyed.

The young temple priestess, Cassandra, denies the sexual advances of Apollo, and so is condemned by him to forever know the truth but never to be believed. Even knowing the truth, she is "barren" in the sense that she cannot communicate it. She lives on the threshold between Olympus and earth, participating in both but neither of them. As a mythical figure she tells us that intermediate realms between mortal doubting and immortal truth will always remain ambiguous. The Delphic Oracle, an actual woman who prophesied in riddles and was interpreted by priests to querants on behalf of city states and royal figures, still leaves us without the surety of truth. Both the mythical maiden and the state oracle show that human beings live in a state of knowing and not knowing simultaneously, and that there are always riddles and paradoxes in our lives. They also show us that the riddle and the quest to solve it are equally important, because it is our natural desire to experience wonder even as we seek answers to profound questions.

Myths are also full of stories like Semele's, the mother of Dionysus, who asks Zeus, her lover, to show her his true nature. Since he has to abide by his oath to the river Styx to give her whatever she asks, he accedes to her wish but with deep reluctance, because he knows it will destroy her. His revelation of his authentic being as a lightning bolt rips Semele to pieces and she burns to the ground. Such revelations, arising from our desperate truth-seeking, inevitably render us lame, blind, or catastrophically blasted into fragments.

Human beings are not made to see gods face to face. We are creatures who live in intermediacies, half knowing, half not knowing. Because of this, we are always seeking and questing. And that is both our creative power and our limitation. We live in riddles and we worship angels.

I am writing this book now because I sense that in our modern attempts to become members of western political and economic life, we seem to have lost our way. The wonder and joy of paradox and the welcoming of ambiguity is experienced by many as an event of deep anxiety.

Many of us have somehow strayed from our deep connections with nature, community, and all else that lies beyond us and within us. We have forgotten that our own psyches are made up of all these elements and that we need to live in empathic relation with them. Early cultures would believe that climate change and disease are the vengeance natural forces take for our somewhat careless dismissal of their presence, for turning them into our slaves and servants out of a certain arrogance and hubris within ourselves that they are here only for us and not themselves. We do not live with them in harmony, balance, and mutual respect.

Rigidifications of religions into their own separate fundamentalisms show us the pulling back of our own arms from embracing others of our own species. Needing to fill the emptiness this lack of relationship causes keeps us from loving, forgiving, and sometimes sacrificing in the face of others' suffering. This attitude keeps us from recognizing the sameness underlying our uniqueness and differences. Not to ask profound, unanswerable questions nor to give ourselves the time to glory in the natural beauty that surrounds us is a way of keeping ourselves armored against both what is within and without. And that leads to feeling empty of nature, empty of the gods and community. Without such relationships, we even come to see ourselves as mere reflections in a rippling pond, like Narcissus.

It is our diviners, shamans, poets, and our psychoanalysts who still believe in healing the human soul rather than simply pragmatically fixing people, as well as those of our scientists and physicists still respectfully open to further mysteries of the unknown who can bring us healing by keeping us grounded and humble in the mysteries of otherness. These are the prophets we need to listen to, because they bring us back to who we essentially are as human beings in relation.

But how do we as modern western selves with egos carefully bound and structured to understand and act successfully within a political, economic world recognize the crucial importance of participating in these liminal, imaginal worlds? In this age of social media and the surface planes of virtual reality, it sometimes feels to me as if our lives have become too shallow, too busy, too thoughtless, to become fully alive and immersed in liminal, complex psychological life. Some of us idealize the notion of creating ourselves as cyborgs and mechanical monsters, because there is no apparent way to exist otherwise.

As a professor at a liberal arts institution today, I am watching the humanities themselves become no longer hallowed spaces for learning how to think philosophically, ethically, historically, poetically, religiously, or linguistically. I fear that they are on the way to becoming mere sideshows for entertainment, mere handmaidens for STEM (Science, Technology, Engineering and Mathematics) and driven to the nether regions by some who teach ideologies to the exclusion of liberal, rational discourse and discussions that can deepen thinking.

It is my hope that sharing my personal experiences, their elucidations in psychoanalytic theory, and my knowledge of archaic Greek views of the psyche through its literary transformations of language in the context of its own sociopolitical development, I will help to further enrich contemporary psychological languages that address transitional and transformational ways of understanding the psyche in relationship. I also hope that ancient Greek scholars will be enriched by knowledge of psychological views of liminal experience as it pertains to their own discipline. I believe that going back to early Greek, pre-platonic, and pre-political ways of understanding the psyche will provide us with a paradigm for recreating our own ways of being intimate with all beings.

Experiencing from a liminal and imaginal perspective is crucial because it is here that personal psychological transformations happen, that genius springs forth and produces not mere repetitions but new ways of perceiving and living in the world. It opens up possibilities for understanding non-western cultures and literatures, in which humans live within the liminal as their primary way of being. Sensing our own integrity in the maelstrom of the world's multiplicity is what will ultimately lead to action, change, and transformation. Perhaps most important, a liminal perspective can reveal to us psychic realms in which we come to experience ourselves as most intensely alive participants in an interconnected world.

Reference

Wheelwright, P. (ed.) (1966). *The Presocratics.* New York: Odyssey Press.

Chapter 2

An Autobiographical Case Study

When I was a child, my imagination became my singular, safe and reliable home. Every time I awakened to participate in the so-called agendas of daily life, I felt simultaneously thrown into the unsettling, fragmenting, and chaotic psychic landscapes of my mother's life and work. She was considered a genius by those who lived around her, which meant to me that I was supposed to forgive her for the tumult of our life and her all too present absence from me. Her pioneering ideas drove her beyond the limits of any single human's capacity to contain and express to the world. She appeared possessed by them at times, as if she was being driven and used by some cruel, Dionysian god. I suspect we both lived with a sense of deep longing and emptiness.

2.1 Helen Flanders Dunbar

Helen Flanders Dunbar (1902–59), BD, MD, PhD, and Med. Sc., received her first three degrees in five years after graduating from Bryn Mawr College. The fourth was honorary. Her belief that specific kinds of neuroses are linked to specific kinds of physical ailments led to her passion for psychosomatic medicine, a field in which she became famous for being able to diagnose and treat mental illness in the interests of physical healing. She was widely known to the lay public for her writing on why people are accident prone, why they live to be centenarians and, somewhat ironically for me, how to understand your own and your child's mind and body. She was also a Dante scholar, deeply imbued with a talent for symbolic thought. She published her

DOI: 10.4324/9781003340751-3

PhD dissertation on Dante: *Symbolism in Medieval Thought*, in 1929, and her most distinguished professional text, *Emotions and Bodily Changes*, in 1935. Both were prominent in their fields and remain so to some extent today.

Helen herself was a fairytale figure for me. She was 4'11" tall and wore size 3.5 five-inch-high platform shoes. She was beautiful in an elfin way, endlessly curious, flirtatious, brilliant, and seductive. Her eyes were an emerald green, set off by her dark hair and olive complexion. They sparkled with intelligence. When she entered a room, her radiance cast others in its shadow. People not only said she was a genius; they said she had "charisma." When I learned that this word was related to other words like chrism, Christ, charity, joy, and grace, it fit my sense of her. She was not only elf, but goddess. Even her medical school male classmates called her "Pocket Minerva." She smiled mischievously when telling me that, as if she somehow held the winning hand.

Women admired her; men fell in love with her; I idolized her. Up to the time that she became almost forgotten, people would smile and exclaim with some awe when I was introduced: "Oh, you're Dr. Dunbar's daughter!" We were a shared identity. I felt like an extension of her body. I poured myself into her and she cast the soft gold of her presence around me. Much later, I discovered that she had been instrumental in setting up the major organization for the training of pastors in clinical counseling. I was contacted by Columbia University to give one of the first of the Helen Flanders Dunbar-endowed lectures to celebrate that group. I gave several talks around the country about her, and I'll never forget an African minister who came up to me after one of them, kneeled down and kissed my feet. I had become my divine mother incarnate!

I learned somewhere along the line that her first published writing was an inquiry into why certain pilgrims who travel to Lourdes experience the miracle of cure and others do not. Later in her life, after I was born, this spiritual side of my mother was something she appeared not to want to talk about, although I could always sense it in her. I remember walking into her New York City office once and hearing her declaim the priesthood for not understanding abortion, saying that if the clergy believed in souls, they ought to learn how to treat them. She said this quite passionately and firmly, which is probably why I remember it. After her death, I read some letters on her yearning for Catholicism – or a higher Episcopalian faith than that of her lower denominational ministerial family. I also found a gold threaded and patterned priest's robe among her belongings, the sort of garment a "low" Episcopalian would never wear. She told my father that her family had disowned her for her higher and more symbolic beliefs and, consequently, had refused to pay for her trip to Europe to study religion and psychoanalysis. She paid for it herself by cutting off her hair and selling it. It was heavy, dark, thick, and fell to her ankles. I loved this story, but always held such tales in abeyance because they were not necessarily true; nevertheless, they were part of the way she became a fairy tale figure for me.

2.2 Childhood

I was born in 1941, when my mother was 39 years old, during her illustrious career and approximately four months before the bombing of Pearl Harbor. My first five years coincided with the beginning and end of World War II, during which time my father was frequently in London writing about the War. He was 55 when I was born. He was a prolific writer, poet, and economics editor of the *New Republic* in its glory days (the 1930s), I thought he was the kindest father – almost grandfather – that ever lived.

My fantasy is that my conception was "a surprise" that occurred on a wildly orgiastic New Year's Eve celebration. I was an only child. My absent father adored me, and my mother seemed to love me and want the very best for me. During our weeks in New York City, where she practiced psychoanalysis, maids and secretaries took care of me in between their cleaning and administrative duties. That did not mean I was not with my mother. I was, in fact, almost always with her, but simultaneously separated either by a door to her consulting room that I was forbidden to enter, a conference in a foreign city, or other professional obligations. From the very start of my life, I felt that my ever present and idealized mother was mostly absent, although I remember once when I was about ten or so, we went to a restaurant together and she taught me how one could discern, by looking at people's facial complexions, expressions, and the way they comported themselves, what they might die of. She wanted to heal them before they became physically ill. She was always focused on preventive medicine. She always insisted on treating the human being instead of the diagnosis.

My parents separated when I was one year of age, and when I was three years old, I found myself on a strange rollercoaster of a life in which my mother and I moved to spend part time in Greenwich, CT to live with a man who proved to be psychotic. I lived in dread of his abuse of her, and as his disease grew more florid, he threatened to kidnap me and kill my father if my mother abandoned him. I remember being snuck out to meet my father in the dead of night and driving with him in our old green Ford truck to our beautiful Connecticut home in the Berkshires. This memory is a fragment and does not fit in seamlessly with others.

Another fragment of memory I have is waking up in the middle of the night to see police lights flashing through my bedroom window in our Berkshire home. I cannot place the date. From what I gathered, my so-called stepfather was running around the grounds outside with a gun and threatening to kill my father. I must have been around five. Or was I eight? Time sweeps and crumbles for me as I think of those years, but I do know that sometime between those two ages, both my mother and I climbed out of her office window in the night, this time with suitcases, to escape my stepfather. These years for me were fraught with sadness, fear, terror, and the emerging sense that whatever was happening was a kind of nightmare. It hardly seemed real.

When I was ten, my stepfather killed himself. That was one of the only times that I ever saw my mother weep. She was standing under the awning of our New York City apartment building when I returned from school, talking to news reporters whom

I believe had just announced it to her. I confess that I felt a huge sense of relief at that time to learn of his death. It was as if all the letters in the crossword puzzle and even the empty boxes swirling about me all those years had suddenly fallen back into place and made sense.

As the world of Greenwich dropped away, I returned to a life of living in the city on the weekdays and spending weekends in the Berkshires. I identified myself with "Merryall," as it was called, because it was finished being built while I was being born. It was always the place I considered to be home. It was the magical place where my father, although still separated from my mother, would join us on the weekends.

Merryall was cared for by European refugees from World War II. Here I could feel the comfort of being mothered by the soft hills, woods, and quiet lakes. The caretakers whom I was later to learn were from such romantic places as Sweden, Germany, Latvia, and Poland, took special notice of me. I look back now and wonder if they felt sorry for me. Edith, who stayed with us longest, taught me to say "eight" in Swedish when I was eight. The number was magical to me because it seemed as if it was a kind of whistling sound turning into a word but not there yet. I loved Edith and made her repeat "eight" in Swedish again and again. I began to trust this space where something was almost beginning to be something but not quite. Edith's husband was equally magical to me because his name was August, and I was born in August. In my young mind, this created a mysterious bond between us. Such people immersed my world in fairytale presences. They filled my head with entrancing and sometimes terrifying fantasy stories that they claimed really happened "in the old country." I lived and played in many countries of imaginary worlds.

My mother liked to tell the story of a German woman who used to cook for us before Edith came. She named the lake nestled in the valley below our home, "The Eye of God." She used to consult it regularly as if it were an oracle. One evening we sat down at the dinner table, and no dinner was served. After minutes of being unable to rouse anyone in the kitchen, my mother went outside and found her on the hill above our home. "Oh, Doctor, I'm sorry," she said, "but the full moon was so beautiful!" Dinners were frequently late because she was outside gazing at the moon. My mother did nothing to discourage this state of mind in either her or me. She in fact encouraged it, telling me once that this woman consulted the "Eye of God" at my birth, asking it my name, and called my mother in the New York City Hospital to tell her almost the very name she had already given me, except, she said, it was missing one letter. She heard the Eye of God say, "Maria."

It was clear to me that my mother had an intuition that bordered on the mystical and the clairvoyant. I think she hid this from the Freudian-soaked atmosphere of New York in the 1940s and 1950s. But it came out one evening when I saw her standing alone on the deck of our country home and went out to be with her. I think I was around 15. We were quiet together, watching the last bit of red and gold slivers of sunlight fade over the soft Berkshire hills. She turned to me, and said: "Winnie (a nickname from my middle name Winslow), if you had the choice, would you rather see half of a sunset or none at all?" Something in the way she said this struck me as odd. It was a rare moment of intimacy, touched by a sense of awe and even some fear, because she seemed to be asking me this as if I were an adult and as if it were a profound, philosophical question. I was not aware at that time, as she was, that she would not live much longer.

For many years, the memory of sweeping colors cascading around the setting sun as day faded into night, and the possibility of there being "half" a sunset as if it somehow stopped in the middle, consumed me. I began to understand the transformative power of metaphor to hold and to express the ecstasy and suffering of human beings.

Long before this I had lived in fairytales that I believed to be true. Being a lonely child and longing for friends, I made myself believe that if I ran outside early enough in the morning, I might look under a leaf and see "Colorkin" (an elf from one of my favorite children's stories) painting the flowers and leaves in their proper seasonal attire. I would crouch down waiting for him to present himself so that we could have talks about important, moral things. But he always eluded me.

I believed that Old Mother West Wind, the protagonist in one of my other favorite tales, was around somewhere with her Merry Little Breezes in a sack on her back. She would let them out to tell her the news of what was going on in the surrounding forests and meadows. They reported to her such things as Skunk stealing eggs at night, in response to which Old Mother West Wind imposed a suitable punishment of painting a white stripe down its back so Skunk couldn't steal without being noticed. Robins, too headstrong and flippant to build nests in the right season, were punished with loneliness, for they could have no children. I especially liked the consequences these animals received. It was the orderliness and justice of their world that made the characters believable for me. I found safety there and perhaps a sense of just retribution.

As I think back on this today, I realize how much I wanted rules and discipline to hold myself together. My mother was a free thinker (she was in her 20s in the 1920s) and she did not wish to burden me with religious, ethical, or moral codes. I became a free spirit but, without discipline, I felt awash in a boundaryless world.

I remember especially the way shafts of sunlight would come in and rest on a spot on the floor next to my bed in the early morning. Even years later, in moments of emptiness and loneliness, I would remember those beams of light pouring in the window and it gave me the energy to stay alive. I feel it today too, when the sun shines suddenly through the shade, as well as in J.M.W. Turner's paintings of Venetian shipwrecks and sunsets.

2.3 Post-WW II Years (1946–57)

I traveled with my mother to mental health conferences in Europe from the time I was five until I was 16. These two-week periods were special for me, as we were together physically a great deal of the time. But my remembrances of those times from 1946–52 are filled with chaotic images of bombed houses in London, deep pits next to strafed buildings, sometimes with pieces of shattered walls still standing. The lovely French countryside was dotted with mere roofs on the ground, inhabited by desolated people. We were invited to stay for a night in a half-destroyed farmhouse where we slept in wet sheets with bedbugs. I remember Berlin especially, a place my mother had loved and known before the war. It had been decimated. This was the only other time I ever saw my mother weep. As I watched her from the back seat of the car, I felt a strange twisting feeling inside that I had never felt before. I believe now that I was experiencing my own heart breaking as I saw her tears.

I recall mental institutions that my mother and I visited where there were still bars on the windows and ECT (Electroconvulsive Therapy) treatments were an everyday affair. Today I can hear as clearly as I could 40 years ago the screams of patients undergoing shock treatment, the wailing of paranoid old men who suffered from what was then called dementia praecox. I can feel the hand of the catatonic woman which came to rest absently on my shoulder to my utter terror, and my mother saying "Just keep walking" as I heard the heavy metal door clank locked behind us.

I remember a dark sanatorium somewhere in Germany, surrounded by trees, on a humid, sultry summer evening, where I was told to stay in a large screened-in sitting room with an old upright piano, while my mother consulted with a well-known doctor. Patients, presumably not so mentally disturbed, sat there in old rocking chairs and on threadbare couches. The air was warm and thick. An eerie, mysterious man settled by my side on the piano stool and told me stories, weaving fantasies like my fairytales but in broken English with a strong foreign accent and an otherworldly air, spinning me further and further into his delusional mind.

I remember being terrified yet also feeling safe in this space. I especially liked the piano. I had played since I was three, and it felt like a friend, although when I tried out a few notes on its yellowed keys, it was very out of tune. When my mother came to pick me up, I was relieved, and yet I had a strange feeling of comfort there, as if I understood already everything about it.

I remember these times as filled with a magical aura. The honor and respect with which my mother was treated made me feel like a princess. Everything appeared to swirl around her as a center, and I was treated as her special and only daughter. Perhaps it was these moments of rare intimacy with a mother who was always close but rarely available, combined with an August day of Zurich sunshine at Burgholzle Mental Hospital, where I met a large, kindly giant of a man, whom I later was to identify as "Dr. Jung." These experiences later moved me into my love of psyche, and especially into the wonders of symbolic process. I was ten years old.

It was a fact that I could not distinguish my chaos from my mother's or from the chaos left by the war. Experiences were fused. Perhaps the major thing I learned as a child was that the world was entirely permeable. Boundaries between me, my mother, mental patients, and what people tried to tell me was objective reality, simply did not exist. Osmosis, symbiosis, swimming paramecia-like in a great semi-conscious sea appeared the only authentic experience.

From about my eleventh to my twelfth year, my mother's life became increasingly troubled and unhappy. I remember feeling unmoored during that time. Part of it was that she became more famous, was working harder and drinking more. Since I was growing old enough to take care of myself, I frequently found myself alone in our new apartment after school, which was now some several blocks separated from her office. Sometimes she didn't come home until late at night.

During these years, I found solace and comfort in reading, among other books, *Alice in Wonderland.* I believe it was my favorite tale because it reflected my own experience. As I read it, I felt myself stepping through a looking glass to find my reflection in a mirror reversed; I became unexpectedly smaller or larger in a house that had looked immense suddenly growing tight and constricting around me and then growing large again. I sat at a tea party of truly mad hatters to find a dormouse asleep in the tea pot. Nobody could pour tea without awakening the creature and that was forbidden. I met a white rabbit with a huge pocket watch on a chain always late for a very important date, except that there never was one. I saw the grinning smile of the Cheshire Cat appear without the cat attached. Stories like this were mad and absurd; they existed in creative spaces at once there and the not there, uncertain, and in-between. Yet they resonated with my own childhood feelings and experiences, while happily enclosed within the covers of a book. I felt somehow recognized. I ask myself now what lured me so to these experiences? Was it the tea party that sounded so delightful, or the dormouse that made drinking tea impossible? The Cheshire cat, or the smile that announced its absence? The white rabbit, or its hastening to arrive at a date that is never there? All of these were just how my life felt – full of upside down-ness, never quite knowing where I was or where I was going, and the inevitable unfulfilled promises I met along the way.

In *Alice Through the Looking Glass*, a much more troubling book for a child my age, Tweedledum and Tweedledee accompanied me on chessboards. The Jabberwocky spoke scary nonsense. The Red Queen with her flamingo croquet mallets and her ringing repetitive words "Off with their heads!" became terrifyingly real, because my mother was quick to fire her helpers, some of whom were people I counted on to set my own head straight.

My mother herself loved riddles and enjoyed Alice. On the rare occasions when we walked together, she never felt I was fast enough to keep up with her, and her voice would suddenly ring forth: "Will you walk a little faster said the whiting to the snail, there's a porpoise right behind me, and he's treading on my tail!" My mother was not a patient woman, and it was a necessity that things go her way. We called her consulting chair her "throne." She was indeed something of a red queen – but a beautiful one.

In Homer's *Odyssey*, which I read when I was 11 years old, there were darker and more emotional and suspenseful moments in the adventures of the hero Odysseus than of Alice, such as when he gets constantly marooned on various islands in great danger of never returning home to Penelope, whether caught by the drenching scent of lotus flowers, the impossibly seductive Calypso, or the underworld itself, where he meets the shade of his mother and tries to grasp her in his arms only to find that she fades away as air. Even as I rejoiced in these multiple adventures and felt the "happy ever after" of Odysseus' return home to the long enduring Penelope, I was later to discover that even that final return was short-lived. I felt a sense of fear, even dread, when I learned that it was not long after his final return that Odysseus is commandeered by a god to journey inland with his oar on his shoulder to a place where its inhabitants have no idea what an oar is and call it a winnowing fan. So much for journeys home at last. I wondered sometimes if there would ever be a happy ending.

2.4 Catastrophe

On the morning after my 13th birthday, we were in a horrifying automobile crash in which my mother was thrown over two lanes of highway traffic and almost killed. She never fully recovered. At this point the continuous fantasy life that had stood me in such good stead during my childhood years began to fail. I was told that I did not concentrate well in school, that I was often distracted and dreamy. When I was at home, I did nothing much, certainly not my homework. At some point, I even stopped reading (these were in the days before television). It seemed that another world had broken in and told me that my own world of fantasy and fairytale could no longer comfort me. I was miserable most of the time. There were group activities I was invited to do which I was too shy and too ashamed to participate in. I was not good at my studies and I was poor at sports. I was a chubby teenager with a bad complexion and had little success with boys. Because I had a professional mother, I was not accepted in a rigid upper-class society that believed mothers should stay at home and care for their children. Whatever the cause, I felt rejected. The only things I did find occasional solace in were music, poetry, and daydreaming.

It was the week before I started college that I found my mother floating face down in the water in our basement swimming pool, dead. Everything went black after that. A heavy curtain seemed to have fallen over my future life. All I know is that I asked the funeral director to keep the leather casket she was taken away in unzipped so that she could breathe properly.

She had said three things to me on that fateful morning, which intruded like vicious animals that I tried to keep at bay. Twelve hours before her accidental drowning, she had been unable to rise. She stayed lying on her own patients' horsehair couch, where she had taken to sleeping. As I sat close to her, afraid and seeing that she was very sick, she said to me, "Winnie, what am I going to do without you when you go to college?" I felt sick in the pit of my stomach. Then there was a very long pause. She turned on her side, looked at me directly and asked, "Winnie, do you love me?"

It has grieved me to this day, over 60 years later, that I was unable to respond. For years thereafter I sat in her chair at the dinner table, slept in her bed, and occasionally wore her clothes, which remained in the closet for years. I changed nothing in our home. I knew I had to live for her. I knew I had to be both of us.

During my first months in college, I had a repetitive nightmare, in which I would see her approaching me out of the ocean, appearing to rise and float above it in a beautiful white gown. I would run to her through the waves and try to throw my arms around her, but wraithlike, like Odysseus' mother, she dissolved to my touch. My roommate told me that I would wake up screaming. I continued to swim frequently, always feeling her mysterious closeness. I did not shed a tear over her death until ten years later. I was 27 years old.

It started one day when I was washing dishes after dinner. The water was streaming from the faucet into the sink. I started to cry into the dishwater. I couldn't stop. That was when a farmer from down the hill who worked in a mental institution for extra pay and who had done odd jobs around our home for many years, suggested I talk to a psychiatrist.

Given the sudden and traumatic loss in my life, it was gradually made clear to me that I was suffering from shock, abandonment, and grief, all of which embody the paradoxical and paralogical. Nevertheless, much of my non-grieving earlier life had actively encouraged a way of being in the world that blurred the imaginary and the real, often in an unobjectionable and saving way.

Children's tales that I had believed and lived in as I explored the natural world, people around me who consulted nature as if it were divine and could give answers, mental patients who provided an intensity of experience both in their fantasy visions and in their unconventional breakings of sense boundaries – all were put back to back with a mother whose fame and beauty held me in a haloed aura punctuated by devastation and absence, and a war and postwar environment that taught me material worlds that looked permanent could crumble in an instant. All this I took in as moments of life – one no more fantastic or dreamlike than the other. Surely, much of it brought trauma, but it was also a privilege, as personal wounds and imaginings mixed with existential losses and wondrous deviances gave me an unusual perspective on the nature of reality.

2.5 Professional Challenges

My college years created a sanctuary as well as a refuge for me. My intellectual interests turned quickly to poetry, and questions of time and the "eternal moment" in Dostoevsky's fiction. I danced and played a lot of piano. To graduate from college felt like falling off the edges of the earth. I wanted to stay forever.

In having to decide what to do with my life, I found myself drawn back to my father's early love of ancient Greek, which he used to quote vibrantly at the dinner table. Those magical moments, coupled with my still unresolved trauma, drew me to enter the monastic seclusion of graduate school, and to become an ancient Greek scholar. Everything I had felt, not wanted to feel and "numbed out" as they say today, poured into my studies.

Not having had much Greek in college, I slept five hours a night trying to catch up to the young male Cambridge and Oxford scholars I was in graduate school with. I had leapt into a different world that occupied every second of my waking life. It was an engrossing, harsh, and powerful escape from my feelings.

The Greek language itself held a highly complex set of structures and rules, which, like French, had endless whimsical exceptions. It is a language suited to riddles, the liminal and the imaginal. It reminded me of the imaginary spaces I had lived in as a child. I loved it.

When it was time to choose a dissertation topic, I found myself lured by the language of oracles. I was fascinated by the way oracular answers were formed and what that might have to do with the relationship that humans had with their gods. I discovered that at Delphi, the so-called navel of Greece, oracles were delivered in riddling form by a pre- or post-menstrual woman in the throes of inspiration. She delivered the messages she heard from Apollo in a kind of crude hexameter verse. The only way to really understand what she said was not to take her literally. Stories about her were legion, but one thing that seemed clear was that communication between gods and humans were ambiguous, mysterious, and seemed to emerge from liminal fields between heaven and earth, and from the very edges of rational speech. This indicated to me that the archaic Greeks believed there was genuine communication between gods and men, but that it was incommunicable and virtually inexpressible.

I then discovered that in pre-oracular times, in the early archaic period when Homer's *Iliad* and *Odyssey* as well as the earlier *Homeric Hymns* had been composed, people read signs that came from a genuine world of gods who lived and breathed between an effervescent and brilliant blue Greek sky, its craggy mountains, "wine dark" sea, and sunbaked earth. Here was an earlier culture that did not have to bring the gods into being, because they already existed! Gods simply looked like larger-than-life humans, although with considerably more power and vision. Gods talked to humans, and humans to Gods. This gave me hope that my own world of fantasy, fairytales, and dreams and my consequent desire to explore liminal and imaginal realms in riddles and oracular language was about something familiar and remembered that had long since been forgotten. These were genuine experiences that I was later to discover Sigmund Freud called "the uncanny." But Freud found a different realm for them, describing them not as living figures in a crystal blue sky, but as emerging disguised from a subliminal, dark, and censoring realm that he called the unconscious.

I began to sense that the transformational symbolic spaces I had become familiar with in my own life strongly resembled what I perceived as the polytheistic and permeable psychic atmosphere inhabited by the archaic Greeks. This atmosphere, as I understood it, permeated a daily, lived world. This was a realm in which humans, nature, and divinities were naturally rooted and intertwined.

That Greek heroes interacted with gods and natural forces as if they all mingled in the same atmosphere also suggested to me there might be lurking in archaic narratives a way of describing and understanding a psyche at once permeable and whole. Archaic Greek narratives of heroes, of interplay with gods, monsters, and signs were not locked in books to be discovered by a single reader, as I had to do, and were definitely not submerged in a dark subterranean world of the unconscious, but were sung and imagined as existing by entire communities across a vibrant, natural, living world. The Greek people lived and interacted with these creatures, not only in dreamscape but in landscape as well. Gods were recognized in the flash of a bird's wing and in claps of thunder. They inspired poets, warriors, dancers, and lovers. Dionysus did not emerge from the chaotic darkness of a tortured psyche to compel the weak into addiction; he danced with his maenads on wild mountain tops, engaging in sacred, orgiastic rites of birth and renewal. Even dreams were understood as visitations from the gods. Querants who visited the temple of Asclepius slept on cots amid temple snakes and dreamed dreams that were then interpreted by the priests of this first legendary physician. Many sufferers were cured of their physical as well as their psychic pain in so doing.

These archaic Greeks lived in the days before the formation of the city-state and even afterward in the countryside. They organized their lives in a highly ritualized space-time framework, where the hearth snake was fed in the morning, acknowledgment was then made to Hermes of the crossroads, and festivals celebrating the various of life's initiatory stages from birth to death were part of a carefully kept calendar (Nilsson, 1940). It was that ritual, tribal existence celebrated amid gods, nature, and the community that later became a more complex culture guided by individual moral, ethical, and political codes.

In later archaic and classical times, such living realms had to be wrenched into meaning through a new kind of thinking created perhaps out of a sense of a felt necessity to separate from the gods, nature, and community. There came about a hitherto unknown interiority of self-consciousness as well as a developing conscience that had to withstand its own fragilities in the increasingly more complex world of the ancient Mediterranean. By Heraclitus' time, and even more in Sophocles', people no long spoke directly with gods. They had to communicate only through oracles, riddles, and dreams. What a huge shift in human consciousness! This is, I suppose, where it all started for me too. But without living gods to see and speak with, I at least wanted to stay immersed in their world, which I could do through attending to the ambiguous, paradoxical language of riddles, fantasies, dreams, and fairytales – the space of the liminal and imaginal.

The world I found in the Classics was an affirmation of what I sensed was a crucial, psychic truth of my childhood. It determined much of my professional life. But after years of teaching about my beloved Greeks, I found myself still driven and restless. I kept feeling a profound desire to become a psychoanalyst like my mother. I became tired of referring my troubled students to others. I felt overcome with the need not just to analyze characters in ancient Greek tragedy, but to treat living human psyches equally driven to discover themselves.

I had been warned by my psychotherapists that to follow my brilliant mother's profession was "pathological" and would be injurious to my struggles to become a separate being with my own desires. But what if I was in fact so like my mother that I had to follow in her footsteps? It felt like a destiny that I could not escape.

I threw myself into psychology and psychoanalytic studies in a second PhD program, adding clinical work based on my studies in Jungian psychology, and contemporary psychoanalytic theories. Here once again I began to discover languages that echoed profoundly my deepest intuition of what it might mean to become a self-directed person while remaining webbed in dreams, fantasies, nature, the community, and all that lies beyond our conscious understanding.

This did not happen without a struggle or without feeling that I too was at times drowning and gasping for air. The trauma I experienced at my mother's death compounded it all and pursued me relentlessly throughout my life. Yet it was precisely working through a fragmented early life ending with this seismic disaster that served as an impetus for me to explore the fluidity of different layers of human psychic experience and to find a sense of coherence in that multiplicity.

As I studied, I found myself riveted especially on the notions of psychoanalytic writers who focus on theories of transitional experience to understand psychic process, and returned to my profession as a classicist, but with new perspectives. I hoped that by exploring and writing about the characteristics of the psyche as it appeared in archaic Greek texts, I might open avenues for richer insights into the human psyche than do contemporary psychological formulations that take as their starting point the necessity of inner coherence.

Liminal and imaginal experiences of my childhood together with my classical studies suddenly became illuminated through the works of these analytic theorists who, although representing many different kinds of thinking in their work, all seemed in one way or another to be identifying a kind of psyche that even and perhaps especially in its fluidity can find different ways to mediate experiences existing on seemingly different levels of reality – levels that appear more or less "real," more or less "conscious," more or less rationally controlled. The chaos of my child psyche, dreaming, fantasizing, imagining, and experiencing unusual and traumatic experiences of so-called reality surely could lead to confused, if not delusional thinking, but also to the creation of great poetry and art. I imagined this psyche as woven together loosely like a Turkish rug, not too tightly or with too much attention to binding the borders. It is said that the weavers always leave a thread that leads to the edge of the carpet so that the soul can escape from the weaving.

References

Dunbar, H.F. (1929). *Symbolism in Medieval Thought and its Consummation in the Divine Comedy*. New Haven: Yale University Press.

Dunbar, F. (1954). *Emotions and Bodily Changes: A survey of literature on psychosomatic interrelationships, 1910–1953* (3rd ed.). NY: Columbia University Press.

Nilsson, M. (1940). *Greek Popular Religion.* New York: Columbia University Press.

Chapter 3

Dreams and Transitional Experiences

Klein, Winnicott, and Kohut

It was between the ages of three and five years old, as nearly as I can remember, that I had two recurring dreams. Both of them were different from the more comforting liminal fantasy realms I have previously described. They had a haunting repetitiveness, demanding to be seen and heard. When I was a child, they always surprised me when they came back to mind. They arrived suddenly, accompanied by traces of dread and disappointment, and I tried to push them away. I couldn't understand them. As an adult, reading about theories of transitional space, the dreams suddenly seemed clearer. Indeed, in reading Winnicott, it was not long before I began to sense that they were all about issues of maternal merging and separation.

In the first dream, I would wake up in the dream to find myself going downstairs to enter a small toy store with narrow wooden shelves rising up to a high ceiling and crammed with every toy one could imagine. The dream was brightly colored but also took place in the shadow. It was an old store, run by a wizened old man. I would stand there, drenched in the joy of color and unlimited stuffed animals, little doll house furniture, and dolls. I could feel viscerally the anticipation of knowing that I could choose any of these toys and take it out of my dream with me. I would always take a teddy bear, hold it fast against me and hope with all my being that when I awoke it would still be there nestled close to my body. It was excruciating to awaken with my arms flat and empty against my chest.

My early and repeated dream blends into a memory of a bizarre episode on Madison Avenue in New York City when

DOI: 10.4324/9781003340751-4

I was on the way home from the school bus stop. I was about eight years old. I had my nose pressed against a toy store window and was gazing at the display. An elderly gentleman appeared suddenly at my side and surprised me by saying: "Do you like toys?" Although I knew I wasn't supposed to talk to strangers, I answered, "Yes." "Come with me," he said, "I'll buy you anything you want." I was drawn in by longing. But I froze with apprehension as I looked desperately and blankly around at all the toys on the shelves. I felt that something was expected of me that I could not do. The teddy bears had to be too expensive. I finally chose the smallest, most inexpensive-looking toy I could find– a little witch puppet with a long nose. "Is that all you want?" he asked. I nodded. The clerk then gave it to me, and the elderly gentleman paid and vanished.

This event happening in reality strangely replicates my earliest dream. In my actual experience, the toy was brought from the shelf and put into my hands. I could take it from the toy store. It was mine. Indeed, a dream come true! But rather than feeling this way, the event was frightening to me and filled with fear and shame. Later, I felt anxious and guilty recalling how crestfallen the gentleman looked when I chose something so small and must have seemed so terrified. Remarkably, I felt the same sense of disillusionment with the actual puppet in my hands that I had when I woke up empty-handed from my toy store dream without my teddy bear. Long afterwards, for I did keep the witch puppet, it aroused in me the most intense revulsion. What happened?

In my second repetitive dream, a nightmare, I would wake up in the dream itself in startled fear to see great black, panting wolves, their sharp-toothed mouths dripping with saliva, leaping through the open second-story windows just in front of my bed and coming to devour me. I would jump out of bed (still in my dream) to find myself running through a vast desert where large machines, like derricks, were digging up huge mouthfuls of sand, presumably in the process of construction. I had frequently peeked through the knotholes in the tall fences surrounding empty city lots, watching these monstrous machines as they dug up the earth in preparation for building. But, in the dream, the background scene was a dark, still wasteland. A single wolf would still be chasing me, and my footsteps would become slower and slower as I sank into the sand, unable to escape. I would wake just before its mouth was on me, in tremendous relief.

The toy store dream faded gradually as I gave up even the vaguest hope of ever having my dream bear. The nightmare I finally resolved by making a conscious decision one night to abandon my desperate flight. I felt the wolf's jaws closing around my neck and allowed myself to be devoured. I awoke immediately, amazed to be still whole and alive. After that, the dream never recurred.

In musing on these experiences, I am struck by a sense of being unable to distinguish between dream and real experience. The dreams seemed quite real, but the actual experience in the toy store (the puppet was really on my closet shelf) felt dreamlike. All three experiences remain far more vivid than many daylight activities I have experienced since. I am also surprised, as I think back, at the distinctness of the dark pathway through which I tried to take the bear from sleep to waking, and the confidence I had that this could be accomplished. I am equally surprised by the resolute decision I made in my nightmare to let the wolf devour me, feeling, paradoxically, as much relief at having done so as I did when I woke up realizing I had escaped the multiple wolves.

If "clarity and distinctness" are enlightenment criteria for what defines reality from dream, then the dreams I had were more "distinct" than the inchoate shadows of my reality. My toy store dream was radiant and bright with energy. It had more substance, more clarity, definition, and texture than anything that occurred in my lonely waking hours. To hold the bear in my arms aa I pressed it against my chest to take it with me into waking … how could it not be really "real"? It brought me a sense of comfort and aliveness that would let me plunge into life overjoyed and safe as if it were still in my arms.

The action itself of carrying the dream bear through the dark path into reality from the dream was perhaps the most alive feeling of all. As an adult, I wonder how the child that had that dream, feeling the sense of complete helplessness and despair as she awoke to find nothing in her arms, had the strength to go on living. Were there any possible living substitutes?

Strangely, it was psychological theories of the meaning of transitional space that in themselves eventually replaced my teddy bear, becoming in effect new transitional objects, and their authors my new idealizable parents. Grasping their concepts and taking them in as part of my own nourishment was like awakening from a dream to find my teddy bear still there. But this was not in the sense of a dream becoming "reality" or actuality. Rather, these concepts had the same sense of the imaginal as did my dreams. They brought a sense of aliveness into the playrooms of my mind, which in themselves felt like the return of a lost mother. A concept, I decided, is something that I could hold onto like a teddy bear and make my own.

3.1 D.W. Winnicott

D.W. Winnicott describes transitional objects as existing in a symbolic, intermediate (potential) space, taking the place of the mother in an extended way and moving the infant from primary merger with her to the recognition of something that she has herself created. This "neither-nor" object, also termed "space of illusion," the baby gives up when she no longer needs it. She no longer needs it when she has internalized the mother sufficiently to feel connected to her even in her absence (Winnicott, 1971, pp. 1–6).

The baby at this point is able to "use" the object. The paradoxical phrase "Hullo Object, I destroyed you. I love you" (Winnicott, *Playing and Reality*, 1971, Ch. 6, p. 8) indicates that the baby can safely play only when the mother can survive the destruction of her most intense affects. "Destruction" for Winnicott is simply a metaphor for the child being able to assert herself without having to fear that mother respond negatively. It is not an aggressive drive in the service of destruction. The mother's ability to stand firm allows the child to play without feeling the anxiety of falling apart. The capacity to play is essential, because, as Winnicott says, “it is in playing, and only in playing, that the individual … is able to be creative … and it is only in being creative that the individual discovers the self” (p. 54).

Winnicott helped me to understand that there exists a space neither “real” nor “unreal” that has a texture all of its own, where light moves and plays through shadows – akin to the experience of seeing sunlight filtering through a leafy shade.

In calling the transitional space a “space of illusion,” Winnicott gifts a double meaning to the word, by playing on its Latin root “to play in.” This grants to it a realistic “thereness,” in addition to its “not-thereness.” Neither dream nor reality, the “substance of illusion” is an intermediate space at once neither real nor unreal, a space where the act of “illusion,” or “playing-in” creates metaphor, which, in its turn, begins to move the baby on a psychic journey to emerge as itself, no longer merged with its mother. It is a crucial stage of growth. By also calling this space of illusion the “root of symbolism in time,” Winnicott means that it is in playing that we discover the possibility of symbolizing, of understanding that things are always more than what they seem. It has, for me, the quality of a flickering liminal and imaginal space, like dreams.

It seemed at first that my desire to take the dream teddy bear into waking was an effort to separate from a sense of being merged with my mother (Winnicott’s phrase “there is no baby” captures this idea beautifully here) and exchange it for a sense of our being each distinct, two rather than one.

Yet, something was missing. Although my dream bear itself might be such an object of transition, I realized that the inability to take it from the dream to make it real suggested that it was not yet existing at the level in which it could represent my own “neither-nor” object, nor was the “space of illusion” comforting. Rather, the dream itself expresses a state of reverie, of mother/infant fusion, and the inability to take the bear (now a part of the dream itself) from the dream indicates a rupture, or the interruption of a more primitive process, that is, an *earlier* developmental deprivation of the presence of the mother, precluding the possibility of providing a transitional object function for me.

The bear that was here but then suddenly vanished as I tried to make it (and so me) real, seemed to express the impossibility of ever separating from my mother. I was left empty-armed and without a sense of my own reality in her absence.

I continued my search for an answer that might reflect what I can only describe as a feeling of empty hunger and found that Winnicott speaks of yet an earlier stage of maternal deprivation. In "The capacity to be alone," he says that the capacity to symbolize, that is, to be in the space of transition, cannot happen without a prior capacity "to be alone in an immature state" (Winnicott, 1957, p. 217). He delineates this preliminary state as one where the infant develops a capacity to be alone in the presence of someone, where "the ego immaturity is naturally balanced by ego support from the mother" (p. 217). In this psychic location, the mother is reliably present "even if represented for a moment by a cot or a pram or the general atmosphere of the immediate environment" (p. 217). The cot or the pram provides a remembrance of the mother's containment.

As I read about these two different psychic locations, both of which consider a symbolic part object as a mother support to enhance development, I mused on what the difference might be between a "cot or a pram" mother symbol, and a transitional object. It seemed to me that the transitional object described the symbolic possibility of genuine development of self without the presence of the mother, leading to the discovery of the child's self, whereas the symbolic part object of the pram is but "a temporary bulwark against nothingness … a protection against the dreaded possibility of what Winnicott calls the "x+y+z moment" (Winnicott, 1971, Ch. 7, p. 97). In this location, the infant can withstand moments x plus y of the mother's absence, but finds that in the z moment, it cannot hold on to its own sense of continuity of being for the length of time the mother is away. It feels "traumatized" in the absence of "mother support." Unfortunately, the mother's eventual but too late return cannot change this altered state:

> Trauma implies that the baby has experienced a break in life's continuity, so that primitive defense now becomes organized

> to defend against a repetition of "unthinkable anxiety" or a return of the acute confusional state that belongs to disintegration of nascent ego structure.
>
> (p. 97)

Part objects, then, like the pram or the cot that stand in for the mother support can be at best temporary and are essentially different from the actual transitional objects that serve as the child's mode of transportation out of the mother's circle of care.

That this symbolic dynamic all seems to be occurring within the dream itself adds a further complexity, because the dream in and of itself is felt as a merger with the nourishing maternal presence. Leaving the dream behind, and not being able to wake up with even the bear as a part object symbolizing the mother/dream merger may lead to a sense of annihilation. Winnicott remarks that a child who has experienced this state has experienced "madness," which mean a breakup of the continuity of existence.

Because this dream experience ends without soothing, comfort, or the bliss of being surrounded by mother, I now understood that my child-self trembled on the verge of annihilation, which in its worst manifestation leads to a loss of desire itself. If this occurs, there is then no availability for the liveliness found in creative playing. This seemed to accurately describe my waking state in that I did possess toys to play with but I could not play. There seemed a deadness about them; neither they nor I could come to life.

It is perhaps this sense of annihilation that led to my second recurring dream of being chased and finally devoured by a wolf. Giving up in despair and allowing myself to be eaten provided me with a huge sense of relief. The dark and haunting quality of an unprotected child roaming the streets of New York City and peering through knot holes into chasms where buildings had stood, to watch great derricks plunging their teeth into the dirt and ruins of buildings, transformed into the lonely desert of the dream, where I was in terrible danger of wolves pursuing and wanting to devour me. In this dark and dangerous atmosphere, finally giving up and allowing the wolf to eat me was also a palpable relief.

What I begin to understand in retrospect is that this act of allowing myself to be devoured represents at once the desire to be merged back into the mother, and a fear of going on living because one is not strong enough to go it alone. In the story of little Red Riding Hood, the disguised grandmother is actually a wolf with "big teeth." Red Riding Hood herself escapes, but the story intimates that the consequence of being devoured has devastating effects because it prevents the child, who inevitably desires to live on her own and to develop her own sense of playfulness and life in the world, from doing so. My dream of letting the wolf devour me implies that it was easier just to allow myself be resorbed by my mother. In other words, my "escape" from terror and trauma was to enter what Winnicott calls non-going-on-being.

What I learned from these dreams, as seen through a Winnicottian lens, revealed more to me about my reality than any of my actual experiences. Looking for a mother-merger would haunt me for most of my life. It would take years of therapy to release me from its power. However, the dream and the inability to make my fantasy bear real, an inability to negotiate a necessary transitional experience from mother fusion to some form of independence, also revealed something else: the depth of my hopefulness. In the dream, "reality" is pictured as an abundant and overflowing toy store. Life is pictured not as depriving but as full of possibilities. I hoped beyond hope that the bear I chose could be real. But what is most real is the hope, which has sustained me over the course of my lifetime.

This understanding moved me to reflect on my actual experience with the kindly gentleman who bought me the toy. Why would I not choose a teddy bear so that my dream wish could actually be fulfilled? Why would I feel so terrified to finally have a toy from the shelf that I could walk out the door with? And finally, why on earth would I choose a nasty little witch puppet?

The dream experiences had been filled with anticipation, joy of discovery, followed by loss and annihilation. But this experience with the kindly gentleman was shrouded with terror. Perhaps the witch puppet I had chosen might be the symbol of a mother who enraged me because of my own deep need for her care in her frequent absences. The witch puppet was a limp cloth of a body dangling from an angry, accusing head. It seemed a part of me and within my control insofar as only my hand could move it or make it come to life. But to do so scared and repulsed me. I hated it and hid it in the dark of my closet where it stayed for years. What had happened?

Winnicott might say I was suffering from an unthinkable anxiety, defined as a felt lack of the continuity of going-on-being because I had not had the mother support to develop the capacity to be alone. Winnicott compares his notion of unthinkable, disintegrative anxiety to the anxiety Melanie Klein defines as "annihilating," or "persecutory" (Winnicott, 1958b, p. 417). This comes from the sense of the mother as absent and so a "bad object."

3.2 Melanie Klein

It was Melanie Klein, in her intrapsychic way of speaking, who appeared to me to capture the complexity of my psychic state more exactly. Klein's language embodies the feeling of being so disintegrated by one's own rageful feelings in response to a mother's absence that the child then projects them into the mother and feels persecuted by her. The witch puppet in this more intrapsychic view of projection and introjection symbolized both my absent mother, who became depriving and hateful because of her absence and by my own "witchy" rageful response to my situation. The witch puppet symbolized my own internal reality, and so I was compelled to choose it! This choice, for all my regret about it, was in fact deeply right, for I unconsciously chose to face reality rather than to cover it over. My world was not only a world of teddy bears, but also witches, and apparently something deep within me had given me the strength and fortitude not to hide from it.

Winnicott and Melanie Klein together form a grand symphony of language by richly attending to what is intrapsychic, interpsychic, and interpersonal which, in my own understanding, enlarges the notion of liminal space. Klein's intrapsychic world expresses the emotional state of the monstrousness of inner psychic objects throwing themselves back and forth in a night-marish world of fusion and confusion, of splitting, projecting, and introjecting, landing finally in an ambivalent realm of mourning, where one "pines" for the "good" part object of the mother, lost as she becomes the "whole" mother containing both good and bad.

Winnicott, holding the intrapsychic together with the inter-personal, adds his own revolutionary understanding of an actual mother providing an actual maternal environment for an actual infant. We could posit that neither intra- nor interpsychic connections are intrinsically relational because they occur in a rather solipsistic way without taking into account an actual self and an actual other. We could also imagine them as internal even as they describe interpersonal connections.

Just as Winnicott wrestles with the idea of internal and external, claiming there can be no self or even origination of self without there already being a sense of inside and an outside, a self and another, there can also be no valid theory based only on a criterion of separation and growth away from the mother that is solely interpersonal. The intrapsychic and the relational are always mixed and intertwined. Both interconnectedness and intrapsychic dynamics exist in a third field that surrounds us, is within us, and in which we are together. Notions of time and space are therefore continually shifting and changing. They are elusive. They are perceived in the liminal and imaginal but only as swiftly moving potentials. This is part of the confusion that I experienced in trying to discern illusion from reality in these early dreams as well as in the bizarre event to which I earlier referred.

The wolf dream as well as the toy store dream show what happens where there is a failure of psychic development. If there can be no creation of potential or liminal space, then there is no formation of metaphor, and no psychic journey toward the self, suggesting that the ability to symbolize is alone what allows the psyche to come into being, and without that there is no relation-ship either with self or others. Liminal space, the place where symbols live, therefore, constitutes a crucial third field that unites and envelops the new self and other in relationship.

I was acutely aware of how my experiences of my mother's early and inconsistent absences could well be explained by Klein's and Winnicott's theories. Nevertheless, having worked through their essential ideas, I felt that there was something essentially missing in their theories. I found myself returning to my own liminal experiences with fairytales, stories, fantasies and dreams so rich and fulfilling that I rebelled at the idea of discovering myself only in a developmental stage between mother fusion and finding my own self as separate. It all seemed quite constraining. My own experience felt quite different in that the very "fantasies" in which I had lived had already woven me into a fabric of words and stories that formed their own space and ground. I felt that they had already created a language of self-healing by softening actual traumas that I experienced with my mother in early life and then settled into imaginal realms that formed one complex and integrative pattern.

That I came to look at dreams through a psychoanalytic lens at all suddenly seemed preordained from my childhood. It was a revelation for me to realize I had felt comfortable with the language of "psychoanalysis" almost from the moment I understood words. I felt as if I had grown up with it as a native tongue.

Again, this was all about my mother, who included and excluded me in her professional life in unusual ways. For one, she always thought out loud and dictated her books, sometimes in my presence. Her eyes sparkled as she talked out her ideas at the dinner table and driving with her to our Connecticut home. During those times, I was captivated by the light in her eyes. Her happiness was my joy. I believe that it was in this way that psychoanalytic theory became a kind of sustaining maternal environment for me.

3.3 Heinz Kohut

This experience suggests that my dream experiences were telling me something about how my response to my mother's actual presence and simultaneous absence became an integral part of my own understanding of the nature of liminal and imaginal psychic space. It suggests that Kohut's famous phrase, "the gleam in the mother's eye," which is above all what gives the child the capacity to feel nourished, expansive, and also promotes self-motivated activity, may not have to be directed at the child herself, but that it can be achieved through the mother's delight in her own insights and intelligence, which then seeps into the daughter to build her own sense of pride and self-assurance. In amplification of Kohut's ideas, perhaps "the gleam in the mother's eyes" for her own ideas might make her daughter feel affirmed as well, carrying its own specific nourishment and ambition with it. If so, this suggests a third field through which "transmuting internalization" occurs – a liminal space that can transmit its own idiosyncratic maternal substance that is then transformed into the daughter's own. Kohut says that one's primary selfobject experiences are as vital as oxygen to self-formation and we can somehow metabolize those experiences into our own protein to build an individual self. Perhaps we need also to add that sometimes what is transmuted can be a shared set of talents and skills, developed not only genetically, but acquired precisely through the gleam in the mother's eyes at her own insightful discoveries, which then get internalized by her daughter. There is very little that made me feel happier than to see my mother happy. It was the sheer taking in of her joy that filled me and gave me confidence.

Kohut asserts the necessity of both the idealizing and the mirroring transferences in the healing process. He tells us that it is inevitable for a child to find that her necessarily idealized parents on whom she depends for survival itself will fall off their pedestals and that the child will then have to create her own ideals (Kohut, 1966, 1971). But what if the daughter discovers that her mother is already famous, already idealized by all around her, and feels from her earliest conscious moment already gathered up into her mother's shining world?

When my mother dictated her books, the words and the gleam in her eye for creating ideas was part of my own sustenance. I idealized her and mirrored her both at once. She felt that I was part of her. I felt that she was part of me. It was not her gleam alone for her special daughter who was a part of her that counted, but our fused gleam for each other. I caught the beams of her words shining in the sunlight and was warmed by them and, since I was her daughter and a crucial selfobject for her, we reflected each other. We basked in one another's glow. I was held in the cradle of the fullness of nourishment the gleam in my mother's eyes could give me as she gazed off in the distance, captured by her own extraordinary insights.

One might suggest here that liminal and imaginal experiences always contain transitional phenomena as described by psychoanalytic theorists, but insofar as these phenomena are considered transitional in nature: that is, insofar as they have a goal of creating the infant as a subject apart from the mother, they are demanding further development of us from merging to separation. They are telling us to leave behind our cherished transitional objects to pass into a new stage of a more distinct and separate sense of reality. Even if development always retains traces of the past and occurs in coalescing and shifting geological layers, there is still a forward thrust, still the expectation of linear development into separation over time, which may ultimately be blinding us to our own desires for remaining in the transitional in the very midst of forward change, that is, the desire to carry our mothers with us no matter what. What if the child always participates in the self-selfobject relationship with the mother and forms a continuously fluid relationship?

One might also ask why separation and individuation are even seen as essential features of maturity. This idea arises from a modern ideal of self-sufficient individuality that is deeply connected with having to maintain an independent ego in order to live in a civic and increasingly capitalistic environment. In comparison to Winnicott and Klein, Kohut's concept of growing into maturity does not involve the idea of separation, but of a healthy narcissism imbued with increased empathy, creativity, humor, acceptance of transience, and wisdom, all of which keep us highly connected with others and the world. Admittedly, merging is a form of identity-sharing that has no possibility of interconnectedness, because, as Winnicott says, "there is no baby," no "other" to relate to. Nevertheless, taking individualism as far as we have in the western world overlooks a relational interconnectedness of great intimacy and involvement that no longer feels like separation or "individuality." It is all interwoven. As Marian Tolpin observed with her customary acuteness, the teddy bear is not left behind once the supposed successful separation from the mother occurs, but remains with us sometimes well into older age (Tolpin, 1976). We never outgrow our need for a relational home.

References

Kohut, H. (1966). Forms and transformations of narcissism. *Journal of the American Psychoanalytic Association*, 14: 243–272.

Kohut, H. (1971). *The Analysis of the Self: A Systematic Approach to the Psychoanalytic Treatment of Narcissistic Personality Disorders.* New York: International Universities Press.

Tolpin, M.M.D. (1976). On the beginnings of a cohesive self – An application of the concept of transmuting internalization to the study of the transitional object and signal anxiety. *Psychoanalytic Study of the Child*, (26): 316–352.

Winnicott, D.W. (1957). The capacity to be alone. International Journal of Psychoanalysis, 39: 217.

Winnicott, D.W. (1958b). Primary maternal preoccupation. In *Through Paediatrics to Psycho-analysis* (pp. 300–306). New York: Basic Books.

Winnicott, D.W. (1971). Transitional objects and transitional phenomena. In *Playing and Reality* (pp. 1–25). London: Routledge.

Chapter 4

Transpersonal and Transformational Space

The Archetypal Great Mother and the Maternal Idiom

New potential spaces connecting now with my earlier liminal experiences appeared to open beyond the personal and lead to a kind of spiritual ground, a recognition of the desire for the fullness of being itself.

As a child, nature had spoken to me in its own vibrant language. Every animal had its own idiosyncratic articulation, from the soft sound of deer hooves stirring the leaves beneath the birch trees, to the lullabies I felt in their gentle, liquid eyes, to the Eastern blue jays squawking me awake in the morning. The golden tones of the rising and setting sun embraced them all. These experiences opened up a space far beyond the personal revealing a world that I felt I participated in but that came from beyond me.

This sense that I was surrounded by an all-enfolding maternal nature had little to do either with transitional objects that were supposed to move me from being fused with my mother to becoming separate and able to "use" her. Nor, indeed, did I feel I was struggling in a Kleinian world of intrapsychic objects in conflict with one another struggling to become a whole from a split and paranoid/schizoid position.

Rather, I sensed that all was permeable; all creatures flowed in and out of one another while maintaining their own particularity. How different this felt from being an objective observer looking out conceptually at the otherness of the world!

Nature, I thought, must be ensouled, and I am one of its many parts. Its surface shimmers, beckoning me to a depth that lies within it. Nature calls to me as if I am a stranger, yet

DOI: 10.4324/9781003340751-5

something in me recognizes that we are one. Here there is no struggle in discerning reality from dream, because all is alive and distinct – a living actuality. Fantasy alone might have driven me within myself to isolation, but now my psyche opened out into deeper meanings that had already been holding me without my knowledge.

I believe this might be like the experience of the archaic Greeks, in which metamorphoses from human to plant, tree, or animal and vice versa were felt as real experiences. In this ancient world, dreams were not called creations of our unconscious minds, but understood as sent by divine messengers to tell us what to do and how to negotiate a wider, more fluid cosmos. All these forms in nature for the ancient psyche, as Harrison says, "tremble(d) on the verge of personality" (Themis, 1962b, p. 67).

My own horizons were opening beyond the personal. I was coming to sense that the human psyche can access universal and transcendent meanings that sustain hope and offer unrecognized depths of experience.

There were theorists, as well, whose sensibilities to nature, the sacred, and the mythopoetic resonated with mine because they had, it seemed, found themselves in similar psychic places.

4.1 C.G. Jung

C.G. Jung, in whose work I had immersed myself for many years, anchored his theory in the notion of a collective unconscious made up of archetypal universal patterns. Archetypal patterns express themselves in particularized cultural forms. but ultimately express such human experiences as birth, initiation, death, the maternal and most especially, the human soul in search of itself.

In his work on nature and soul, Jung says:

> So far as we can see, the collective unconscious is identical with Nature to the extent that Nature herself, including matter, is unknown to us … In my opinion the collective unconscious is the preconscious aspect of things on the

> "animal" or instinctive level of the psyche. Everything that is stated or manifested by the psyche is an expression of the nature of things whereof man is a part.
>
> (Jung, Later Thoughts II, para. 540, Sabini (ed.), 2008)

> What is miraculous in the extreme is that man can have conscious reflective knowledge of these hidden processes, which plants, animals and inorganic bodies seemingly lack. Presumably it would also be an ecstatic experience for a radium atom to know that the time of its decay is exactly determined, or for a butterfly to recognize that the flower has made all the necessary provisions for its propagation.
>
> (Jung, Collected Works II, para. 447, Sabini (ed.), 2008)

Jung exposes a collective space beyond the personal, believing that the human psyche can access universal and transcendent realms of meaning.

4.2 Erich Neumann

The Israeli psychoanalyst and mythographer, Erich Neumann, expanded many of Jung's ideas in his studies of comparative mythology (1973). Neumann tells us that the symbiosis of a human mother and infant is expressed universally as an experience of being held in the surround of a "Great Mother," a variation of which is found in almost every creation myth around the world. This cosmic maternal surround is imaged cross-culturally in its earliest stages as the *ouroboros*, or snake who eats its own tail. Without limbs, or organ distinctions like breasts, stomach or genitals, it forms a perfect circle, providing its own eternal nourishment. It symbolizes not only the ultimate cycling of birth and death, but the womb of the cosmos itself:

> There was something formless yet complete,
> That existed before heaven and earth;
> Without sound, without substance,
> Dependent on nothing, unchanging

All pervading, unfailing.
One may think of it as the mother of all things under heaven.
(Tao The Ching # XXV, tr. A. Waley in *The Way and its Power*, Neumann, 1973, p. 9)

In this circular image, the sudden and harsh demand of having to breathe on one's own when one is taken from the mother's womb need not occur, because feeding and breathing both take place in a sea of symbiotic plenitude. In this symbolic language, the personal is set in the surround of Jung's archetypal, collective unconscious, itself a holding maternal space, not yet even gender-differentiated. It expresses the sense of being both born and remaining unborn simultaneously. Here, my childhood experiences of fusion and separation through potential space open to a world that can be at once merged and distinct, libidinal, yet mysteriously sacred (cf. Neumann 1973, pp. 10–13).

The collective mythic realms of Neumann's archetypal world resonate with and encompass the personal but are not in themselves personal. Adam and Eve's exile from the Garden of Eden because they ate of the forbidden Tree of the Knowledge of Good and Evil is a cultural story specific to the Hebraic tradition, but it can be symbolically understood as the universal expression of the loss of a paradisal world through developing self-consciousness. It is called archetypal because it describes a highly significant experience that is felt by all human beings. Every culture has its own story about paradise.

Such myths embody in their various cultural manifestations the sense of universal human suffering in being wrenched from an innocent and original world through the gaining of consciousness or, in Neumann's words, the loss of the bliss of the oceanic feeling as the blossoming sense of our own consciousness turns back to perceive it. Our very sense of perceiving separates us from it, and we cannot recall the sense of once being one with it without feelings of melancholy and nostalgia.

Stories such as this appear to recall a universal experience that lies even beyond consciousness. In so doing, they evoke a sense of wonder and numinosity ... a sense of being deeply understood by something larger that borders on the mystery of faith. Stories such as this continue to exist and give meaning despite contemporary scientific understandings of earth's origins, which in themselves spawn new myths.

Opening our psyches to a realm of universal meanings that are available to us because we are all members of the human species grounds us in a collective unconscious that reflects the myths and theologies of all peoples. Myths help us to send our roots deep into a common soil to grow a deeper sense of understanding and home in ourselves and with others.

Some of us resist a faith in archetypal and collective realms, considering it a form of pathology. Yet, the only thing "pathological" about understanding our personal psychology through such mythical stories may be the unwillingness or refusal to recognize that the integrity of our own experiences is intertwined and made richer through understanding that something within us finds itself deeply in touch with nature, gods, and community. Perhaps this is because we can't stand losing the sense of self-control and autonomy that tends to accompany the empirical roots of some scientific understandings.

Neumann in his mythical and archetypal language corroborates Winnicott's early stage of the mother/baby unit ("there is no baby") by defining the infant as an "ego germ" that needs to separate from its symbiosis with its "Mother" to develop into a "Hero." Neumann also echoes Klein in his mythological verification of the struggle and rage experienced as this separation takes place. When Neumann uses the archetype of the Great Mother to explain who we were as infants and how we come to be as selves, he shows how the so-called "ego germ" rests in the maternal, basks there, and has no desire to individuate.

But when the hero (ego) emerges, he must begin to separate from that gentle all-encompassing, seductive, womb and move on. This is captured in the myth of the hero Perseus and the Medusa. Looking at her directly, Perseus would be caught and "petrified" by her – scared and turned to stone. But if he can see her reflected in the shield of Athena (goddess of reason and wisdom), he can decapitate her not by looking directly at her, but at her reflection. When he manages to kill her by looking into Athena's shield, this is a symbolic expression of achieving something "through reflection" (the power to become a self-conscious, thinking being) (Barnes, 1974). Decapitating Medusa "through reflection" is a double entendre. It tells us that by being able to engage in reflection, Perseus is no longer merged with the maternal and all it represents, and can view Medusa as an object. Medusa, once a beautiful priestess of Athena, pays the punishment for her rape by Poseidon in Athena's temple by being transformed by her into the snaky-haired woman that we are most familiar with. But the reason for this is not that she is herself evil, but that she herself is so seductive and alluring to men. If Perseus looks on the mother directly, he is tempted to return to her and not continue to develop. She is dangerous only because of the power of our desire to return to her. Rape is no more than the force of desire to return to the mother (which in a patriarchal society renders her subjugated, without subjectivity, without voice (Cixous, 1976).

This myth expresses more than just a personal developmental stage from infancy to ego consciousness; it also affectively arouses in us what it feels like to become human. It evokes a spiritual and existential state of the loneliness of the human condition itself that reaches far beyond the purely personal and yearns nostalgically for a larger maternal home. It provokes a sense of having once been part of an all-encompassing sacred, maternal presence.

Some of us engaged with the study of transitional experience find it uncomfortable to move from the psychologically personal world of subject and object to that of the spiritual and archetypal world where these feelings exist at a cosmic and mythic level. Neumann himself criticizes Freud for his personalizing erotic idealizations of the mother figure, suggesting that [for him] sexual desire lands only on the personal mother, when what we actually desire and long for is an original, fully nourishing and all-encompassing mother that holds us all in her embrace (p. 14).

Neumann is a Jungian with whom we might begin to soften the boundaries between psychoanalytic and Jungian analytic theory, which are frequently seen as irreconcilable because of their ideological differences. But object relational psychoanalysts like Michael Eigen, Christopher Bollas, and many others also use language that is not closed to what we might call the sacred maternal and may be seen as bridging Jung and Freud.

4.3 Michael Eigen

Michael Eigen suggests that there is a realm that is "prior to and beyond Kleinian introjective-projective dramas" (1981, p. 413). He says: "My immediate concern is the way object usage takes the life of faith in transitional experience forward" (p. 416). Faith for Eigen is "a faith in a spontaneous play of experiencing and meaning which aims to express and unfold what is most real for the subject, "his emotional truth or way of being a subject, who one is" (p. 431). This faith is always in complex tension, because it has to recognize itself in a third field of creativity and mystery beyond the certainties of time and space.

If, as Eigen suggests, transitional experiencing is about faith in spontaneous play that reveals who we are most fundamentally as subjects, then longing for reunion with the cosmic mother (or god) cannot be a mere substitution for the loss of the personal mother, nor can turning to the sacred to soothe our feelings be merely a function of our needy emptiness – a mother substitute, if you will. Attaining a sense of one's own reality always occurs within and beyond time and space certainties, at the "intersection of profound vulnerability and saving indestructibility … that brings the paradox of faith to a new level" (Eigen, 1981, p. 416).

Neumann and Eigen both strongly suggest in their writing that liminal and imaginal fields stand on their own as crucial for the human psyche. If, indeed, there can be health and stability in continuing to live in transitional experience, then it itself must inhere in a coherent space where dreams, fantasies, interpersonal connections, and daily events can seem equally real, clear, and intense without the subject's feeling either closed off from connection with "reality" or in an amorphous space of chaos and disintegration (cf. Bromberg, 1998).

4.4 Christopher Bollas

Christopher Bollas, despite being an object relational psychoanalyst, extends Jung's and Neumann's ideas. In his understanding of what he calls transformational space, he brings together the archetypal, the personal mother, and the maternal sacred. In expanding Winnicott's idea of a facilitating maternal environment to that of a transformational maternal idiom, he describes a sense of going-on-being that most echoes my own experience.

What is essential about Bollas' work is that unlike Winnicott's transitional object, it escapes the boundaries of linear time and seems not to put much store either in the developmental line of a relationship required to move from subject (mother/infant unit), to object (the ego separated from the mother and able to "use" objects), or from oneness to twoness.

Bollas understands the transformational experience as a continuous state that expands through amplification rather than developmental time. For him, the future is always discovered through the past. Future contains past, and past, future: "Transformational object seeking is an endless memorial search for something in the future that resides in the past" (Bollas, 1987, p. 40). So, one is never an isolated subject with a particular character standing alone but rather a subject/object forever emerging in relationship and expanding outward, rather like ripples in a pond.

Although Bollas and Winnicott appear to be similar in that the transitional and the transformational experience both occur within the intermediate space of creative playing that Winnicott introduces, the transformational experience that the mother has originally provided is exactly what the infant continues to seek and amplify. "The memory of this early object relation manifests itself in the person's search for an object that promises to transform the self" (Bollas, 1987, p. 2). It is this very search for a transformative experience originally provided by the mother that drives one forward. This may appear paradoxical, as in order to move forward, one must be able to find objects that bring the person back to the infant's experience. The fusion that was once felt with the mother returns during one's involvement with playing creatively or engagement with aesthetic experiences. Each of these offers a chance to re-experience the emotions felt when they were one with their mother by bringing them into the present.

Together with the continually expanding maternal idiom comes an originally experienced sense of reverence, which is "more of an 'existential' than a 'representational knowing'" (1987, p. 14). "Thus, in adult life, the object is pursued in order to surrender to it as a medium that alters the self, where the subject-as-supplicant now feels himself to be the recipient of enviro-somatic caring, identified with metamorphoses of the self" (p. 14).

The sense of a subject-as-supplicant praying for transformation is part of this sense of experiential reverence that Bollas describes. Such reverence leads in adult life to the search for transforming aesthetic experiences, experiences that can only be felt through the language of symbol, metaphor, and narrative story.

Bollas describes this experience using the story of Water Rat in the (well-known) children's book *The Wind in the Willows*. Water Rat awakens one morning as he and his companion, Mole, are rowing downstream, and Water Rat is startled by "an ethereal sound" (Bollas, 1987, p. 38).

> "So beautiful and so strange and new," he says. "Since it was to end so soon, I almost wish I had never heard it. For it has roused a longing in me that is pain, and nothing seems worthwhile but just to hear that sound once more and going on listening to it forever … rapt, transformed, trembling, he was possessed in all his senses by this new divine thing that caught up his helpless soul and swung and dandled it, a powerless but happy infant in a strong sustaining grasp."
>
> (Bollas, 1987, p. 38)

Bollas calls this experience "uncanny" because, paradoxically, it is not the unfamiliar that helps growth, nor a sense of standing alone apart from the mother, but a recognition of a reverential, transcendent sense of being that one experienced long ago in the sustaining grasp of the mother. The "familiar" mother idiom is necessary to experience the new "unfamiliar" growth (transformation). The future lies in the past. Past and future are recognized together in the reverential and transcendent moment of transformation and carried forward in an ever-expanding psychic landscape. It is these moments of what Bollas calls "the uncanny" that we are always seeking, be it in a symphony, a sunrise, or one's own writing.

Winnicott doesn't speak of creative fields of play emerging from the early sense of being one's own character, nor does he go so far as to say that it is the desire for transformation itself that moves one forward. But he comes close to what Bollas will explain further when he says: "in the world of the unit self the subject grows through the continuous cycle of putting self in others and others in self" (Eigen, 1981, p. 416).

For Bollas, the idiosyncratic ego (or character) is already embedded in the infant. Self-consciousness is inherent. Bollas says it is embellished as a result of the mother's interactions with the as yet nonverbal child, the songs she sings it, the lullabies, the way she holds the child, and so forth. Good-enough mothering is the ability to "manipulate the environment to make it correspond to human need" (p. 36).

Bollas' world describes a kind of dreaming by day where our psyches are unconsciously choosing evocative objects to use as dream material in the days and nights ahead: "We are living out a kind of unconscious aesthetic … a perception, a thought, something overheard is noticed and then transformed by an exceptionally furtive artist" (Philips, 1994, p. 156).

Bollas' aesthetic language calls up states of mood, of the uncanny, of a music that invites us to enter the liminal and to discover ourselves in a living idiom of our own being. Images are unconsciously evoked to thread us between the spaces we stand in. This experience, which Bollas defines as the aesthetic idiom, is where the speakable and ineffable meet. When we stand in between the spaces of our self states (Bollas, 1987, p. 46), we experience and speak from this idiom. Thus, when Bollas says that "we learn the grammar of being before we learn the rules of our language" (p. 46), he is voicing a poetic sense of what constitutes who we are in our ineffable being before we learn how to speak it to ourselves. When he says that the sacred precedes the maternal, he is speaking of the sense we have of our being before we are even aware of the maternal idiom, which is the predecessor and carrier of our later aesthetic experience.

Bollas describes children's literature as "replete with moments of horror, awe, fascination and suspense … where self and environment are mutually transformative, as if something of the child's sense of ontogenetic metamorphosis is registered in the fiction he reads." Poetry, Bollas thinks, presents to the child's psyche the possibility for growth in its own being. In *The Wind in the Willows* the wonder is vividly expressed in Water Rat's experience of sensing the sunrise. It is a transcendent space present in its very absence, "felt," through "ethereal sound." This third field of intermediate presence evokes a space of reverence. Bollas reminds us of Neumann when he says:

> It is possible to see how the reduction of spiritual experiences to the discrete administration of the mother always strikes us as somehow an insult to the integrity of uncanny experience, since "*the sacred precedes the maternal*" [my italics]. Our earliest experience is prior to our knowing of the mother as an object in her own right.
>
> (p. 39)

Returning to my experiences of mother-longing and loss in dreams, I recognized that the dream about the toy store had its own reverential, transcendent feel. It promised transformation, but then because of a terrible gap and discontinuous nourishing, I fell into a schizoid position, "*where language is dissociated from feeling, and where the moods of the internal world are almost exclusively rendered in the subject's way of being*" (Bollas, 1987, p. 37, my italics).

Bollas' language is fraught with a longing to return to the maternal idiom, but also to transform that idiom, carrying the particular sense of the maternal idiom forward in more expansive ways. If, as he says, "the sacred precedes the maternal" and is transmitted through the mother, then the longing for the mother must also must also contain a longing for return to the earlier "sacred" space that precedes the mother.

My early autobiography and the dreams that accompanied them now appeared to gain more clarity. It seemed that to be whole and healthy I must embrace transformational experience; however fraught it was with longing. Bollas' words were nonpathological, and appeared indeed to lead to an acceptance of the human condition.

The work of Christopher Bollas brought the numinous and its archetypal resonances first understood by Jung and Neumann into my understanding of self and world. His aesthetic language and radiant symbols carried me on paths through which I arrived at a sense of the transcendent, which filled me with wonder, and the sense that I was part of something beyond me, part of a whole. I felt that nature, the divine and the human community all are animated by that connection – even stones are drawn together through their magnetic power – even bronze breathes.

C.G. Jung opened for me the field of a collective unconscious, and Neumann flooded it with culturally particular myths that symbolize archetypally significant patterns. Bollas helped me to absorb these patterns through his mythopoeic use of language. All three authors awakened me to the possibilities of the transpersonal and the transcendent, liminal realms that I felt were crucial for achieving the depth and fullness of individuation.

I now see that my attempt to understand myself through the theories of others was in itself an act of searching for mirroring insights and yearning to be held as a child in their theoretical cradles. Feeling understood by their theories was akin to being held by a mother, perhaps herself clinging to theories that she then was able to advance as part of her own perspective. Perhaps she had also felt herself coming to be a creative self through their potential and nurturing spaces.

Reading Bollas on the transformational object was transformational for me. The longing for an often-absent personal mother in itself led to my sense of being held by psychoanalytic theories acting as mothers. But the actual discovery of home came about through the recognition that I could move within the maternal idiom in a circular and expanding dance throughout my life.

The sense of home happens precisely in this transcendent moment of recognition, of the "uncanny," as Bollas says, in which one becomes known to the other, and the past returns to the present, ever circling and amplifying, yet also ever the same. Here is the magical clarity and simplicity that we all yearn for – that all be known, understood, and made familiar in its very expansion, felt as illumination and the presence of mystery simultaneously. Home is felt here as an ever familiar yet expanding destiny.

The language of transitional space as used by Winnicott, the cosmic, mythic language of Neumann, and the mythopoeic language of Bollas are all describing in their own ways permeable liminal and imaginal realms. It is precisely the aesthetic, creative, and empathic languages in which all these authors write about how the child feels as it moves into its own space from the mother's arms that were transformative and transmutative for my own psyche.

These writings helped me to feel at home in myself and in liminal realms, which in their illusive but substantial nature express the fluid reality of all the objects we meet throughout life. Living through these spaces, for me, was like living with the angels, or within the angelic realm of the Sufis, or Plato's ultimate sea of beauty in the Symposium ... all expressing the anticipation of salvation through the presence of absence.

The liminal in all its aspects seemed to be life itself. Finding ways to express it so as to keep it alive seemed to me a task of immediacy and necessity. But this was impossible without some semblance of self-structure.

In an impressionist painting, this structure is achieved through the boundaries of windows and paths. These are the open and breathing spaces one imagines seeing and walking through. They allow us the frames to immerse ourselves in all the complexities and mixtures of color and soft shapes that seem to pour into one another. But it is the colors and flowing shapes that are center stage, and the windows and paths are only needed for the sake of seeing and wandering through the colors. Imagine the lady in the garden of many impressionist paintings who cannot be recognized as different from the multitude of flowers in her garden, except by the hint of the parasol she is holding, and yet she is the essential center of the piece, as one imagines her perceiving the scene.

Emotionally, I had actually felt at times as if I were immersed in the fields of a Monet painting or the rushing cacophony of colors and jittery brush strokes of a Van Gogh. My own psychic environment, dwelling in the space between fantasy and dreaming held the texture of a spider web. A spider spins its world out from itself. The thread from its spinerettes creates its own home. Although seemingly infinitely fragile to an outside observer, my web provided me with a strong and elastic habitat; It simply wove everything into itself by expanding its boundaries. There was always a secret hidden here, a mystery that would give me the final answers. My whole life was a search for origins, for the origin beyond all mysteries.

But, after my mother's sudden drowning, skeins of this web had begun to rip apart and become unsustainable. A new and imperative voice sounded forth, proclaiming that the magical spaces of the liminal and imaginal fields that had kept me safe with my gloriously present and absent mother in childhood were, for all my wishing, suddenly insufficient. I had now to confront the abyss made hopelessly real by her all too sudden, tragic, and irredeemable death.

References

Barnes, H.E. (1974). *The Meddling Gods: Four Essays on Classical Themes.* Lincoln: University of Nebraska Press.

Bollas, C. (1987). *The Shadow of the Object: Psychoanalysis of the Unthought Known.* New York: Columbia University Press.

Eigen, M. (1981). The area of faith in Winnicott, Lacan and Bion. *International Journal of Psychoanalysis* 62: 413–433.

Harrison, J.E. (1962b). *Themis: A Study of the Social Origins of Greek Religion.* Cleveland: Meridian Press.
Jung, C.G. (2008). *The Earth Has a Soul: C.G. Jung on Nature, Technology and Modern Life* (ed. M. Sabini). Berkeley, CA: North Atlantic Press.
Neumann, E. (1973). *The Origins and History of Consciousness* (3rd ed.). Princeton: Princeton University Press.

Chapter 5

Radiance, Mourning, and Creativity

5.1 Melancholia and Radiance

My mother's sudden death had changed my world. The empty wells I had tried to fill by taking on her identity, wearing her clothes, sitting and sleeping where she sat and slept were failing me. Even the liminal worlds I had earlier delighted in were not enough to soothe me. They froze into ice fields, punctuated by raging storms of anger that would descend upon me suddenly and unpredictably.

I covered all of this over with a sense of irreverence and sometimes hysterical and erotic playfulness. My college friends and I dressed in my mother's clothes and held wild dancing parties in the living room of my country home. I am sure these events seemed odd, if not bizarre, to them. But for me, they were shot through with a certain radiance – a mood that I was later to learn Melanie Klein defined precisely as that "radiance that falls on the shadow of the ego" in melancholia (Segal, 1964; Freud, 1917). Beneath these charades of grandiosity and performative antics lay a ghastly abyss of desperation and longing.

Why was it that my dwelling in liminal, imaginal spaces no longer sustained me? Images from my childhood and in my dreams seemed like museum pieces behind glass, ossified. It was as if they were trapped in freeze frames, cranked out in jerky, distorted ways with little narrative, like old silent movies. I felt I was bumping up against them, tripping and falling over them in the dark. Was it the trauma of my mother's drowning that did this?

DOI: 10.4324/9781003340751-6

I became captivated by Freud's idea that in melancholia we identify with the object we have lost, because we cannot bear to lose it. Tragically, it is held in ambivalence by us, partly because of its very abandonment of us through death. Consequently, when our ego identifies with these lost objects, it is also altered by identification with them. The ego then comes to hate itself as it did the lost object with which it has identified. Freud also talks about cannibalizing the lost object by swallowing it whole and then being unable to metabolize it. Neumann's image of the *ouroboros*, or snake that eats its tail, sprang to my mind, as if my mother and I were coiled into each other, mutually swallowing each other, feeding ourselves on each other's empty pain.

I became consumed with the notion of psychoanalytic objects – transitional, transformational, evocative – as various psychoanalytic theorists use them. I was fascinated at how physical and discrete they seemed. They reflected my own sense of being broken into pieces. The emphasis was on the objects. They were not "subjects" that could relate to one another.

Melanie Klein speaks of internal intrapsychic objects in exceptionally concrete ways. In her description of the paranoid/schizoid position, the object of the mother splits into a good breast and a bad breast and must be seen as a whole mother object for the infant to develop her own sense of wholeness. But for the good and the bad to be held together as a whole, the infant must become able to tolerate ambivalence, which evokes a sense of "pining" for the purely good mother breast that is now forever lost.

My feeling of mourning was similarly split. There seemed to be no possibility of moving or growing. Nothing came to life. Beverly Zabriskie (1997) refers to "frozen accidents" (p. 25), spaces of trauma in which fantasies freeze the psyche, not allowing it to play symbolically or to entertain paradox (cf. Winnicott, 1971, Ch. 2).

Melanie Klein has been much criticized for this language of "psychic objects," as if they somehow inhabit in an anthropomorphic but robotic way the physical insides of our bodies. Yet this is just the way traumatic grief feels – as if one is taken over by inanimate monsters not related to oneself or to one another. In this space of freezing and fragmentation Klein's intrapsychic objects made all kinds of emotional sense to me.

James Grotstein (1997) embellishes Klein's language by saying that "whether located externally or internally, the object per se is always a montage, a pentimento, a palimpsest of multiple layers of images" (p. 52). He goes on to say that the original subject of the mother whom we presumably internalize is in and of herself an "individual," and as such is "ineffable" and "unknowable." Put simply, "the pure object" exists only as an hypothesis in virtual reality" (p. 52). Objects are much better seen as changing and complex personifications, creatures, and images of our imaginal worlds. Grotstein draws us out of Klein's terse dialectic of objects, seemingly spoofing it by moving it into this language of monsters. For him, psychic objects are demons "multifariously constructed." "The term monster," he says, "accounts for the gallimaufry assemblage of cannibalized parts that contribute to the grotesque, misshapen bizarre others that characterize these demons" (p. 54).

Grotstein's language resonated with my despair by giving form to the veritable living monstrosities that controlled me as they flickered in and out of my clouded psychic world. But, like Grotstein's comparison of such figures as sealed in the enclosure of "a procrustean bed," or Dante's devil frozen in hell, my plethora of part objects maintained an unfortunate and suffocatingly fixed pattern, even in their moving fragments. They appeared at their most ghostly to cover up the dread of annihilation, chaos, and absence.

Language becomes artful when it describes emotional states exactly as they are felt. When that happens, emotion can begin to flow again. When the verbal description becomes a perfect mirror, such that the experiencer can say "that's it! that's exactly it!" one can begin to feel fully known, fully understood. The artful words of Grotstein affected me emotionally and gave me a sense that I might begin to heal.

For many years reaching out for help had been impossible for me. I felt that my psychoanalyst mother expected me to be a paragon of mental health. It felt like a betrayal of her to admit that there were seams and cracks in my psyche where, if explosive rages burst through, I would be exposing her as a failure. I needed to let everyone know she had raised a perfect child. I had little idea at this time that what I was experiencing were grief reactions to her death exploding emotionally into my everyday life. But I knew I needed to come alive again if I were to function in the world.

My psychological studies were beckoning me to engage with actual human beings. I have spoken about being held intensely and warmly by Winnicott's and Bollas' theories of transitional and transformational experience, as if they themselves substituted for my lost mother's care. It was these theories that finally brought me to trust that there might be actual people in the world who could help me.

5.2 Two Psychotherapies: Classical and Winnicottian

5.2.1 *Dr. B.*

The first psychologist that I was referred to was classically oriented. He helped me to connect my fragmented parts into a narrative. Immensely helpful as it was to feel myself as a subject beginning to feel connected in time, it felt like the wrong story. His was the tale of a highly oedipal child who worshipped her father and was highly enraged at her mother. To this day, I remember Dr. B insisting on my bringing the first copy of my mother's famous book, *Emotions and Bodily Changes*, into his office, tearing it apart, throwing the pieces into the fireplace and watching it go up in flames. Later, the memory of destroying this precious document cut me to the core. The wounds had scarred over, but beneath there was a sea of pain. Dr. B. helped me to overcome my explosive anger by telling me that it was split off and not a part of me, but I concluded after this treatment that the piecing together of personal history through interpretation in psychoanalytic treatment is rather similar to an archaeologist searching for and collecting the shards of a broken tablet scattered and buried for eons in the desert. Even joined together, the pieces never form a coherent whole.

Perhaps Dr. B himself felt as if he were under a set of rubrics that he was uncomfortable with. Like a good analyst at the time, when I invited him to my wedding, he refused. So, I brought him a piece of wedding cake, and when I handed it to him, he wept. I saw him for about four years altogether, and he did much, despite all, to help me to become whole enough to be a caring marriage partner to my second husband.

5.2.2 *Dr. G.*

It was about three years into the marriage that my then seven-year-old daughter from the earlier marriage became suddenly terrified one night that spiders were crawling up and down her legs. At that time, I did not, as I should have, attribute her symptoms to the kitchen fire from the stove that very same evening that was hard to put out. Instead, we took her to a therapist who specialized in families and children. After seeing her for a couple of sessions, he told me she would be fine, but then, with a trace of a grin, said he thought that I was the one who could use some help. Perhaps I seemed to him overly anxious. It was clear to me that I was still feeling as if I needed some healing. He reminded me very much of my deceased father, whose absences when he was alive were far less important to me than the care and love I had felt from him when he was present. I accepted Dr. G's judgment and became his patient.

My father transference with Dr. G. doubtless had to do with the fact that I was replacing my daughter. He did not seem entrenched in any theory, but his manner was Winnicottian. His demeanor was gentle and kind and gradually I began to feel soothed by him as would a small child. Whereas I was drawn to Dr. B, who was quite relaxed and friendly, his manner was somewhat more confrontational and caustic than Dr. G.'s, and I was highly sensitive to that.

Not surprisingly, the liminal, imaginal spaces I had experienced in childhood began to come alive again within me and

I began to feel stronger. I felt the beginnings of a sense of wonder and liveliness, of enhanced creativity.

The creative impulse in a wounded self cannot emerge without a sense of safety and holding. It may birth itself in Nietzschean splendor with a sense of breaking boundaries and moving into an ultimate freedom of spirit, but it needs to begin in deep quiet, a sense of reaching through eons of space or of floating in a still pond and being held by warm, silky water. At least this was what I felt … that the primary act of creativity needs to emerge from a sense that one is at rest and being soothed. If that feeling is not there, and there has been too much trauma, then the creative act itself becomes its own painful and all too often contorted and inauthentic search for healing. At least this was my new story and what I felt was a more truthful narrative than my previous entrapment in an oedipal tale.

Dr. G.'s ability to calm and soothe me fostered dreams that deepened and evolved over our time together, a period of close to ten years. Most of the therapeutic exchanges with him emerged from these dreams to form a third field in the transference that fostered in me a deep longing for self-expression (cf. Winnicott, 1971, Ch. 2, 1965a, pp. 73–81). The key to it all was the joy of mutual playfulness and discovery, of having an affirming, listening presence to be with me on the journey. As I grew stronger, I could reach out through these dreams to connect with others.

I dreamed at the beginning of this therapy of cars strangely plunging *uphill* from the highway in the near distance and threatening to destroy my home. When I told Dr. G. this dream, he said, "I think that you do not feel a strong sense of self." The simplicity and directness of his statement was comforting. I felt an instantaneous sense of hope and calm.

As time went on, I believe that the multiple and playful self that I was eventually to discover came through this holding environment, fundamental to the specific, empathic, therapeutic stance of Winnicott and those who are self psychologically informed. Rather than focusing on rage and oedipal issues in an attempt to interpret my past, Dr. G. immersed himself with me in a pre-oedipal space of play, allowing me to experience the transitional spaces that I had missed and gradually to become conscious of them. I recalled that Winnicott himself characterized analysis as "highly specialized form of *playing* in the service of communication with oneself and others" (Winnicott, 1971, Ch. 2).

Part of the joy of this "*playing*" touched areas of shame and defense over their erotic nature. My therapist was able to calm my anxiety over sexual feelings for him by telling me that they were only felt as sexual because I was now mature and that they were a consequence of overlaying adult feelings on childhood adoration. He said that he wanted me to feel as fully as possible the magical and enchanted adoration that my father evoked, with him.

The feeling of release that this permission brought evoked a projection of all the feelings I needed to be allowed to feel for my father onto Dr. G. (cf. Ornstein, 1980, p. 141). At this time, I dreamed of bearing a husky, robust child, as well as dreaming of Dr. G. with eight nostrils, four ears and four eyes, two of which stared down "golden and glowing" from his eyelids. I wrote soon after that in my journal, "I feel an overwhelming sense of child-love for Dr. G., as if he were my father. I feel as if I am with a real person," and not much later: "Our substances seemed to leap across the room and to embrace" (Personal journal, Dobson, 1984). I believe that the multiplication of his eyes and nostrils in the dream into a kind of golden and alive Hindu god was a dream manifestation of my idealized desire that he might have the ability to know me completely.

My eventual feeling of coming into myself rather than feeling merged with him came in a dream in which I was trying to be "bold," and hiding a "fat and swollen 'change' purse" in various places where it would not fit, finally finding a safe place for it only in my own bureau drawer. As sexual as Freud might find the metaphor, as he had with Dora, and as it perhaps in part was, for me it also indicated the beginning of the "swelling" of the true self and its potential for change. I was hiding it because it indicated a separation from my mother, with whom I had felt I had to stay merged and keep idealized, perhaps even as a "compliant self" (cf. Winnicott, 1965a, pp. 148–150).

This dream of a swollen "change" purse was followed by the therapist's introduction of the image of my psyche as a train moving through a heavy snowstorm, the snow blowing off as it pushed through the winter night. I picked up his imagery in another dream in which I was driving a heavy black sedan through a winter storm. I could not get it to go up a hill, when a small puppy appeared, attached to the front of the car by a clothesline, and pulled the car over the hill. This dream seemed to indicate my ability, through internalizing Dr. G.'s imagery and transforming it, to become my own guide. The symbol-making power, that is, the ability to become creative and to allow dreams to guide me, was an indication that I was beginning to replace my melancholia with mourning.

Hanna Segal reflected my feelings exactly and seemed to sum up this therapy:

> Every aspect of the object, every situation that has to be given up in the process of growing gives rise to symbol formation. In this view, symbol formation is the outcome of a loss; it is a creative work involving the pain and the whole work of mourning. If psychic reality is experienced and differentiated from external reality, the symbol is differentiated from the object; it is felt to be created by the self and can be freely used by the self.
>
> (Segal, 1964, p. 63)

After years of therapy, I was finally able to begin the process of uncovering the rage and tears surrounding my mother's death. At about this time, I took a vacation to Hawaii, where my grieving became intense, and where I ventured into rough waves with an undertow that brought me close to drowning.

Ignoring the warning signs on the beach, I plunged into the swollen surf. I am a strong swimmer, yet the undertow was fierce. But it didn't feel at all dangerous at that moment. Rather, I felt I was plunging into my mother's arms, which the warm, strong undertow, as it dragged me back and forth, reflected. I felt no difference between myself and the waves and I was tempted, as

I felt my body losing strength against them, just to let go and to go under. When I was thrown by a wave back onto the sand, I arose dripping and in what felt like a trance.

That afternoon, my husband, who was with me, and I went to an exhibit at a neighboring hotel put on to benefit the marine life in the area. I browsed through the inevitable and interminable pictures and sculptures of whales and dolphins, when I suddenly saw in front of me a circular bronze relief, about 40 inches across, of the Volcano Goddess Pele (see book cover). Her eyes were closed, her hair, formed to resemble streams of black lava, swirled around an exquisitely serene buddha-like face. In her hand was a torch of blazing fire and surrounding her the artist had crafted flames of polished bronze. She was simultaneously fully masculine and fully feminine, fully enraged and fully serene. Some survival instinct that had willed me away from my desire to feel fused with the ocean waves brought me here to look upon the bronze face of the goddess. Feeling myself merging with her face, I suddenly fainted.

Part of what I thought I saw in Pele was my mother's face. But the healing element of the bronze was that Pele, the epitome of rage and destruction, was here joined with a dreaming serenity. She was conceived as a circle of lava and fire, male and female, shadow and light, with closed eyes and an enigmatic smile, the extremes of her destructiveness and love flowing together in harmony. At that moment, I knew both my mother and myself. The hidden ambivalence which split me unconsciously became whole in my consciousness through this work of art. The flowing together of the different forms of bronze was immediately healing to me.

I believe that throwing myself into the waves was a final desperate attempt to merge with my mother, Afterwards, when I came face to face with the bronze sculpture of Pele, I blacked out. This was a transformative experience because of the aesthetic nature of the sculpture, which embodied my mother's dual creative and destructive nature and my own, in idealized and substantial form.

When I spoke of my experience to Dr. G., he asked me to bring in a picture I had taken of the sculpture. He was struck with awe as he looked at it and said: "It looks just like you!" His empathic affirmation of my own intense response to it moved it into the realm of what Winnicott would call "object use," an ability to use the other and to recognize oneself as subject. This is what Bollas might call a "transformational object," an experience in which the early maternal idiom is present in a transformational form. It was now, when Dr. G. acknowledged and deeply affirmed my own experience of the sculpture, that I was able to see and to integrate my own loving and hating relationship with my mother and to harmonize the ambivalence in myself.

With Pele, I had experienced the power of a maternal, transformational idiom, an aesthetic, reverential moment in which we feel "an uncanny fusion" with the object. Such an event Bollas believes re-evokes an ego state that prevails during early psychic life" (Bollas, 1987, p. 16). He argues that because the mother is transformational for us, we continue to search for that which can transform. It is the process of transformation itself that the mother passes on to us that Bollas believes evokes reverence, creativity, and desire for life.

It wasn't long before I began to feel as if a huge weight had been lifted from my shoulders. For the first time I felt I could breathe by myself. I was free to engage in the substantial and transformational quality of the imaginal world. Here I could welcome multiplicity and the intense reality of dreams. But I could also be present to events as they happened outside in the world because the boundaries between inside and outside had become supple and permeable. It was as if the frozen, fragmented world of fantasy that had at first shut me away from living experience had opened out into a place of fluidity of experience where I felt comfortable with change. More than ever, I felt connected with multiple presences within and without. It was the connections themselves that brought me a sense of wholeness.

5.3 A Self Psychological Analysis with Ernest S. Wolf

Twenty-five years after my second psychotherapy, my 25-year-old daughter gave birth after 26 weeks to twins. I was on sabbatical in Chicago where she lived, thinking I would write a book, but found myself instead with her and her husband at the NICU (Neonatal Intensive Care Unit) of the University of Chicago hospitals helping to take care of two tiny little infants, each of whom weighed a pound at birth, and could fit into the palms of our hands. After almost a year of care, it was clear that the lungs of one would not develop. His brain stopped functioning from lack of oxygen and I watched my daughter and her husband let him die. It was during this time that I entered my third therapy, a self-psychological psychoanalysis.

This time I mourned for my tiny grandson, and even more for my daughter. She keened all night at his passing. I had never heard that strange, wrenching sound before, nor have I since. It evoked the death of my own first child, a daughter, 26 years earlier, who had mysteriously and senselessly died in my uterus nine days before she was born. I thought I was over that. But my grandson's death reawakened it and left me shattered.

At this time, I had myself become a clinician, and was deeply immersed in self psychological theory. I was also a professor of ancient Greek. I had been seeing patients for ten years, and had 16 years of psychotherapy. I thought I was managing and was highly reluctant to enter a third psychotherapy until my husband, seeing me descending into a fragmented and dissociated state, asked whether there were any psychoanalysts in Chicago that I might really desire to work with and learn from. I had never had a genuine psychoanalysis and of course the longing was there … to be on my own mother's couch.

Having read Kohut and Wolf's "The disorders and treatment of the self: An outline" (1978), and Wolf's *Treating the Self* (1978), I said jokingly, having assumed that Dr. Wolf was dead, that I would like to see him. My husband encouraged me to look him up anyway, and to my great surprise I found him on the reference list of the Chicago Psychoanalytic Institute, still quite alive and wanting to see patients. The joke was on me.

Dr. Wolf invited me to come see him the very next afternoon. He was 82 at the time, and we worked together until he was 90. At 97, he died, a dear friend. He opened another world for me, a world of meaning, integrity and structure that has allowed me to write this book, and finally to become an agent of my own creativity.

My analysis with Dr. Wolf with its focus on self structure was unlike my earlier psychotherapies. In the early days of the analysis, I presented to him the world of fairytales, fantasies, and dreams that I depended for vitality and meaning, as well as my passionate professional engagement with ancient Greek language, thought, and literature.

But he seemed strangely uninterested. He seemed to think that because I had recorded my dreams with no focus or connection to my daily life that they left something to be desired. He seemed to think that what might give me a stronger sense of self was to be found elsewhere. I thought later that indeed perhaps I was trying to impress him with my imagination and life as a scholar, the way a child shows a parent her first scrawled pictures and construction paper cut outs. I was disappointed.

But he was right. As we continued to work together, all my fantasies began to seem more like viscose translucencies – glazed windows that I couldn't quite see through. Dr. Wolf brought me to a sense that there was a clarity of vision that I had not previously experienced, landscapes and cities lurking beyond my clouded vision, shimmering out of my reach. Walking with a sense that my feet were on the ground, rather than floating through an insubstantial reality gave me a sense of simple and clear view of objects that I had formerly found too traumatic, and definitely uninteresting. I learned that my dreamy reflections radiated off of concrete things. Houses, churches, cobblestones, winding streets and so forth were not just in fairytales; they actually existed. He taught me that when I put my feet down from this dance of fantastic reflections, there was a floor to land on. He taught me I could trust that – even enjoy it. But most surprising to me was that rather than consider all the other possible avenues of grief we could explore, he focused on only one, from start to finish.

5.2.1 Process in the Analysis

Dr. Wolf was silent during most of our first session, listening to my responses to several gentle queries about my life history.

After a while, he suddenly asked: “Are you sick?” Not knowing what he meant, I was silent. “You’re not sick,” he said, adding, “You’ll feel better soon.” He sounded like a soothing mother. I felt calmed and yet somewhat taken aback. What was he really saying? Was I not worthy of treatment with him? Did I need to be sick? Wasn’t I interesting enough? His warm smile and gruff but softly accented German voice told me otherwise. I wondered later whether being sick was in itself a disguise to protect me from my grief. Or was it that my mother always cared when I was sick, but spent most of her time with patients, so I had to be “sick” if I wanted to see her? Almost as if he had been reading my unconscious thoughts, he loudly and explosively burst out towards the end of that first session: “It’s all about your mother!”

That night I had a dream:

> I am going down a long winding hill to a large mill pond with a house next to it occupied by a couple. At the bottom of the hill, smack in the middle of the road there I see a large dog. It is alive, but instead of having hair, its coat is a thick quilt of bright patchwork designs that zips up its back. I look beyond the dog to the pond I realize I have to cross, which now has a large, revolving wooden water wheel. I begin to notice that the edges of the pond keep flooding over with water, and I despair of ever crossing it.

When I told the dream to Dr. Wolf, he startled me with a soft chuckle. But he neither interpreted nor asked for my associations. Used to therapists who were always interested in associations to dream imagery in dreams, I challenged him on this and he said simply and with a gentle smile, “I interpret when I can.”

What was the meaning of this? Surely not that he could not interpret the dream! The effect of the non-interpretation was that the dream sifted into the silt of a deep pool of unconscious meaning. It was only an hour or so later that my husband and I were at a luncheon café and he accidently spilled his coffee. I became fixated at the liquid pool on the table and the drops as they fell on the café floor. I began to feel quite tearful. We went from there to the Chicago symphony. The program was Mahler's Ninth Symphony. At its end, I was sobbing so profusely I couldn't leave my seat. It seemed that I myself had become the pond in my dream that was flowing over its banks and couldn't hold back.

I wondered later if this would have happened if Dr. Wolf had interpreted the dream. My relationship to Dr. G. had deepened in response to his interpretations of my dreams. But something vital seemed to be happening now as a result of Dr. Wolf's refusing to interpret.

I understood perhaps why he hadn't much later in the analysis when I interpreted the dream myself: I was the dog protected with a thickly quilted coat and held together by patchwork. The dog seemed somehow like a stuffed animal, perhaps representing my need to be protected and cared for as if in my mother's arms. I was zipped up, not ready yet to open up, or perhaps even to have my dream opened up. I thought the couple in the house next to the pond represented me and Dr. Wolf. The flooding mill pond represented the magnitude of my grief.

By not interpreting the dream, but connecting warmly with me in the session through his fatherly chuckle of appreciation, Dr. Wolf gave me a bodily sense of being protected and cared for, despite my desire to involve us both in the dream's interpretation. Had he appreciated the dream aesthetically and worked to interpret it with me, it might have taken me right back to my fairytales. In any case, it was clearly this dream that introduced the main subject of our analysis.

The next time I met with Dr. Wolf, the day after my sudden outpouring of tears listening to Mahler's Ninth, I had a strange experience. I stopped at the front of his building on Michigan Avenue before entering, and looked up at the frieze above its entrance. It was glimmering and flashing gold in the sunlight. I suddenly became dizzy and felt as if I was about to lose my balance. When I went into his office and sat on my chair opposite and somewhat to the right of his, the entire room suddenly and oddly tilted to the left. I was terrified but was able to control my voice. "I think I am having a delusion," I said. When I told him this, Dr. Wolf reacted with his usual calm and curiosity. When I returned for the next session, he asked gently if I had any desire to lie on the couch (which was immediately to my left beneath the window!). Inasmuch as my deepest desire was, in fact, to have a genuine psychoanalysis and, secretly, to be my own mother's patient, I felt like a child whose deepest wish had been unexpectedly granted. I got up from my chair, moved to my left, and lay down on the couch. Dr. Wolf said nothing by way of explanation or interpretation, but I felt better, and the "delusion" was gone.

Dr. Wolf never acknowledged that he recognized I wanted an analysis; he simply understood and responded to my need. Later, when I read about his ideas on the similarities between infant/mother and patient/analyst relationships, I saw that he realized that I needed to be in an early merger transference with him, and that the infant part of me needed an empathic, nonverbal response. Despite the fact that I longed to engage in conversations about self psychology with him, he chose to move into an intrapsychic space of infantile soothing with me. The result was that I felt a profound sense of connection with Dr. Wolf. I felt held, respected, and understood for the first time in my life as a kind of equal, despite my idealization of him.

That was the beginning of the analysis. There are four more moments of process that I think are essential for understanding it as self psychologically informed. All of them have to do with Kohutian so-called narcissistic transferences and those that Wolf added, which, while not excluding an overall transference, represent developmental aspects of myself that I had not experienced in my other psychotherapies.

5.2.1 Idealization

I had earlier noticed Wolf's influential book, *Treating the Self*, prominently displayed on his desk. I had been teaching it for some time, and I told him how much I admired the book. He grunted with a sense of satisfaction. In the next session, I continued to praise the volume. His first comment was, "This is going very well, very well indeed!" He seemed to be preening, and I burst out laughing. Then, as I continued to tell him what an extraordinary volume it actually was, and how much he had influenced the world of self psychology, he said, with some mischief in his voice, "If you continue on like this, I shall have to read it!" It delighted me that he experienced my intense and extraordinary idealization of him with pleasure and humor (cf. Lachmann, 2008). His acceptance of my idealization of him began to integrate disowned and disorganized parts of me into my expanding sense of self in an atmosphere of warmth, safety, and eventually, trust.

5.2.2 Mirroring and Twinship

It was not long after this that I caught sight of a little box on Dr. Wolf's table. I suddenly became curious about what was in it. With much hesitation, my curiosity finally got the better of me, and I gained the courage to ask what was "in the box." (I had rolled over onto my stomach on the couch and was looking up at him.) He chuckled, then smiled and said "Shall we find out?" He opened the box, and we both looked in. "Paper clips," he said, pulling one out, "rubber bands," "a thumb tack …" We took great pleasure in looking carefully at each object, for indeed they seemed imbued with a magical aura to me, and I felt that we were discovering some great secret together.

I believe this moment shows Dr. Wolf's understanding that I was at that moment needing an early mirroring transference with him and that, as a result, he engaged in play with me as one does with a three-year-old. Realizing, perhaps, that no one had ever really played with me, he intuitively understood his role. Significantly, he never asked me why I wanted to know what was in the box, which, I believe, would have destroyed the experiential, empathic space we were in. Rather, he chose to explore it with me, and thus to make each one of those paper clips and rubber bands into a subject of wonder and discovery.

5.2.3 *Falling in Love*

As the analysis continued, I was struck and disturbed by a dream that I narrated reluctantly because despite its childlike imagery, I took it to be erotic:

> I am lying here on your couch, and the couch has turned into a crib. I am looking up at little plastic, colorful animals and figures strung above the crib that I can play with. You are floating above the crib looking down at me.

I was silent for a long time. Finally, feeling very uncomfortable, I said, "I think I am falling in love with you."

He said, after what seemed an interminable pause, "I know."

Astonished, I asked, "How do you know?"

He paused, as if not knowing quite what to say, and then gently, with a bit of humor, he said: "I've been doing this for fifty years ..."

I felt both amused and sheepish. But rather than feeling this as a rupture, or being jealous of other patients who had also "fallen in love," I felt profoundly safe working with this remarkably experienced psychoanalyst.

5.2.4 *Reading Through Dreams*

From the beginning, Dr. Wolf's diagnosis was that this therapy was "all about my mother." He always responded to thoughts and dreams that I had about her with force and brevity.

When I eventually told him about my guilt at feeling I was responsible for her death, he didn't speak, as Dr. B. might have, about my homicidal, unconscious wishes. Rather he said, simply: "You did not kill your mother." Later, when I told him a dream about my mother drowning in a lake outside my window, he said: "Your mother was overwhelmed." I was struck by the fact that he saw my dream not as revealing an unconscious wish that she die, but rather as something I had observed about my mother but had never been willing to recognize ... the childlike vulnerability and fragility beneath her extraordinary brilliance and fame. After Dr. Wolf's surprising comment, I could feel myself flowing with forgiveness and empathy. This deep recognition of my mother's own suffering and overcoming led to a sense of empathy for myself as well, which left me feeling more whole and more at peace.

Very late in the analysis I had a dream in which I saw my mother dying and sinking to the bottom of the swimming pool where she had actually died. She then miraculously rose to the surface, alive again. But she was no longer my mother. She was Dr. Wolf.

When I told Dr. Wolf this, he said in his simple, disarming way: "I have become your mother in this dream."

My mother's death, a week before I turned 18, had prohibited our ever developing a mature, adult relationship. This analysis allowed me not merely to mourn her loss but to experience her as brought back to life through the shared agency of Dr. Wolf and my dreaming self. He had himself become an adult mother to love.

5.2.5 Termination

The analysis was always interwoven with my fear that Dr. Wolf himself would die suddenly. He was clearly living longer than most people have a chance to live. He steadfastly insisted that he was fine and made a point of always being on time for my appointments and being available to me by phone if I needed to speak to him between sessions. But I expressed my anguish about this so continuously that one day with some firmness and, I guessed, underlying frustration, but still with a characteristic twinkle in his eye, he said: "Don't you know that self psychologists are immortal??" And to my frightened question of who I would come to for advice after he died, he said: "You will be fine, because you will know everything I would have said in answer to any questions you might have." I believed him to be right, and it is so to this day. Gradually, I grew to believe that he would indeed survive until the analysis came to a natural end, that he wouldn't die as my mother had, suddenly and traumatically, despite the strong possibility, given his advanced age, that he easily could.

When, after several years of analysis, a few of my analyst friends announced that they were going to retire, I told them that Dr. Wolf had never even raised the question of retiring or even the issue of termination. They were quite concerned; one even suggested that Dr. Wolf was acting out and allowing me to take care of him, which would eventually retraumatize me.

When I reported this to him, he was characteristically unfazed, but spoke with some anger about their judgments. He said: "When you choose to leave, you may come visit me whenever you like – parents don't 'terminate' with their children when they grow up, do they? The relationship just changes."

I believe Dr. Wolf's response showed his belief that it was an absolute, therapeutic necessity for me to rely on him as a parent who would die a natural death in old age, and that he would be with me for the duration.

Gradually, I became more relaxed around the idea that our analytic relationship would end as well as responsive to his offer that I could change our relationship to anything that suited me – chatting ten minutes a week, visiting occasionally – and so forth. When I finally decided that it was time to end our analytic relationship, he was gracious and, I think, relieved. It touched me when he responded, "You are the last person to leave."

I felt a sense of melancholy when he said that, and at the same time very proud that I had been so indisputably precious to him. As it turned out, Dr. Wolf didn't use me before ultimately abandoning me in death. He collaborated with me in an analysis that ended when I was ready for it to end and left me with a sense of wholeness, calm, and coherence which has never left me.

5.2.6 Liminal and Imaginal in Psychoanalysis

Returning to liminality and the importance of imaginal language to engage what is most creative and vibrantly alive in us, one might ask what its function was in this particular analysis. Dr. Wolf had refused at the beginning to join in helping me to read my dreams, nor did he have any reverence for what I felt was sacred and numinous in Jung's understanding of the archetypal, collective unconscious. I had in the early period of our analysis challenged him on that: "You don't believe in it, do you?" I asked. His response was: "Let's just say we both believe in a mystery." He seemed to think that the path to my own psychological growth was for us both to use as little conceptual and imaginative language as possible. I didn't like this, which made these early days of the analysis a winter of discontent. At least this is what I thought then.

But I came to see that despite seeming to reject my fantasies and dreams, he did, in fact, in significant moments, speak in metaphors with me that connected me with him deeply. In these moments, I felt the presence of an intense emotional field between us. He seemed to join with me, empathically understanding my own liminal sensibility.

Out of the blue one day, early in our analysis, at the end of a session, he gazed down from the top floor of his old Chicago office building at the "Bean" then being constructed in Millennium Park, and remarked: "It will be beautiful when it is done." Following his gaze, I looked down out of the window to see fractured mirror segments blazing in the sun, to me, distorted fragments of ugly modernity. Yet, as I recalled this moment later, I wondered whether the "it" in his comment referred not just to the Bean, but to our analysis together. Of course, I don't know, but his words feel to me as if they came from a liminal space, on the threshold of our interconnectedness, and were joining us together.

It was the same when I arose from the couch one rainy day after weeping endlessly. When I reached the door, he said: "You forgot your umbrella. You're going to need it today." In saying this, he showed his empathic understanding of my emotional pain by connecting it metaphorically with the outside rain. It was as if my tears and the tears of the world flowed together and he was gently protecting me. by reminding me, as would a caring parent, that I needed my umbrella. So did he engage us both in third, intermediary fields through which I could take in his empathic nourishment and care. That was indeed what I later understood to be a moment where the metaphorical substance of words allows for the transfer of psychic protein between analyst and patient. Dr. Wolf recognized how I functioned. He recognized me. This in itself was the answer to all my dreams.

5.2.7 Empathy

Empathy, or Einfühlung, "feeling in," creates the psychoanalytic liminal spaces I am describing. It is the energy that flows between and around and within such experiences. It creates a deep and flowing intrapsychic field between two subjects, melting boundaries between them. Sometimes it can give the sense of two souls joining mysteriously in an extraordinary intimacy. It is what Dr. Wolf used to refer to, quoting Virginia Woolf, as "moments of being." It is as difficult to describe how that happens as it is to define the "self." But we know when it is there.

Transference love is a partial name for it – the transferring of deep feelings of love and trust between and within the therapeutic dyad, which always bears similarities to those we have loved, hated, and idealized in the past – those significant people that grew us into consciousness to begin with. That connection in depth leads to still deeper and more transpersonal realms that allow us also to feel connected with nature and with an area of faith that some call "divine," and others simply a cure through love.

Kohut's term for empathy, "vicarious introspection," does not imply the observing, objective eye of the scientist or the doctor. It allows one to sink into a deep reverie through feeling that opens insight into others (cf. Ogden). It is the difference between opening one's eyes right under the surface of an ocean and sinking to the extraordinary world of darkness beneath. That feeling of the mystery of the unknown, yet familiar, is what gradually brings us to understand the other, whoever and whatever that "other" is.

Empathy can be described as communicating through image and using image to open emotionally aesthetic third fields.

Metaphor works suggestively in this space, using words and phrases that mean two (or more) things at once. Metaphors, like riddles, can throw one into a state of wonder through ambiguity. It is this wonder at how the two meanings, so seemingly different, can mean together that one discovers oneself letting go into symbolic intermediacies that are filled with energy and feeling. It makes real a relationship – not only a relationship with one's own imagination, but a felt relationship with another human being. To this day, I recall with a certain wonder Dr. Wolf saying "Einfühlung," in German, and telling me that the literal meaning is "feeling in." When I repeated the word in German, he smiled and said, "You are bilingual." His answer still hovers in the air mysteriously. Whatever it meant, it brought us together.

Dr. Wolf held and became connected with me at the deepest level. I felt I no longer had to weave a spider's web, gathering all to myself. I knew and was hiding it well that a wind, or rain, or a human hand can destroy that supposedly strong weaving at any moment. Being with him for eight years – this tough little old man who looked like a gnome in a fairytale and who had survived trauma far worse than I, yet still had a twinkle in his eye and kind soothing words for me whenever I needed them – this dear friend of Heinz Kohut who loved his family and wasn't afraid of dying, was like a rock for me to climb onto in a stormy ocean. It was in him that I found my relational home.

5.2.8 Wolf's Adversarial Transference

At the beginning, Dr. Wolf, I believe, worked through Kohut's merger, mirroring, idealizing, twinship, and alter-ego transferences with me (Wolf 1978, p. 187). He responded like a parent to my being an infant, then a happy three-year-old. Later he would speak with me quite a bit about Kohut and self psychology, as if I were his equal. But after that, when I felt I wanted just to stay in his maternal nest, he refused to let me, but rather worked with me on spreading my wings and becoming independent.

I always idealized Dr. Wolf. That feeling was the bedrock of all the other developmental moments that occurred. At first, I knew very little about his life and did not know him as a person. But a close interpersonal relationship evolved over time between us. At first, I imagined he was very like me, and I was shocked at the end to discover he wasn't very much like me at all. It came at the moment when I told Dr. Wolf that I had just been to see Götterdämmerung, the last opera of Wagner's Ring Cycle, about the fall of the gods and the destruction of the world, and that I had loved it.

His voice thundered out from behind me: "Wagner? Wagner? I hate Wagner!" His response was so loud and uncharacteristic that I burst out laughing. It wasn't his revulsion for the anti-semitic Wagner with his fondness for the Nazis that made me laugh. It was that by spontaneously sharing his own deeply personal feelings, he made me experience myself as an agent. In that moment, I felt like myself for the first time. Eight years earlier I would have been crushed by Dr. Wolf's hating the composer I so admired. Now, seeing that he and I disagreed profoundly seemed to set me free. But it also brought me to the realization that I had had an effect on him, very much the way Wolf describes how two-year-olds gain a sense of efficacy when they discover they can have an effect on their parents (Wolf, 1978, p. 181).

I found myself writing and publishing more and with greater ease, and becoming increasingly comfortable with my burgeoning life as a self psychologist, where I feel most alive and creative. Even my teaching took on a new sense of exhilaration and vibrancy.

5.2.9 Death

On August 21, 2018, my husband looked up from his computer as we were eating breakfast and said gently: "I have sad news. Ernie Wolf just died." A deep and profound sadness washed over me. I was silent for a long time. I waited to feel traumatized and fragmented. But remarkably, indeed, miraculously, I realized that

I felt neither. Dr. Wolf didn't have to be constantly by my side throughout my life to heal me, and indeed, he didn't even need to stay alive for me. When he died, I didn't swallow him whole, nor did I attempt to cannibalize him as I had my mother. It seemed that little by little I had metabolized the psychological substance he offered me, which consisted largely of his simply being there with me, endlessly patient, unlike my mother, and knowing just what I needed when I needed it. It was this process that allowed me to come into being.

Throughout my analysis with Ernest Wolf, I became eager to read what he had written, and I read everything I could find. In doing so, I discovered that he almost never wrote up a case. When I asked him why, he said it was all too private. I think it was at that time I decided to write up my own analysis with him. I wrote up every session we had verbatim for seven years. One day I walked in carrying in a 5" deep 8" by 11" box that contained the analysis, along with six elaborately covered journals, and put them on his footstool. He looked quite alarmed, and said, "Am I supposed to read all this?" I said "No, but it's our analysis." I asked him what he thought about my writing it up for publication and he said: "Do it when I'm dead."

This shocked me at the time, since Dr. Wolf had always encouraged me to write, and I wrote my first paper in self psychology four years into our analysis (Dobson, 2007). I had felt uneasy about writing in the field and quite sure that Kohut would not like me since I was a classicist. I was, of course, terribly wrong, since the Greeks were a favorite of his (see Dobson, 2020). I felt at that time that the world of imagination that Dr. Wolf had at first rejected in me burst into flower and sent roots into a relational, self psychological world. In any case, here I am, four years later, "doing it when he is dead."

5.4 From Mourning to Creativity: New Versions of Mourning

I have wrestled throughout this book with the substantive, fleshly feel of symbolic meanings that have the power to transform the psyche, and which must, given that we are human, affect the body as well. We are not simply bodies, nor are we only psyches. As humans we experience psyche/soma, in which mind influences body, and body, mind. This is indisputable, although given our western obeisance to Cartesian paradigms, we get edgy in the face of having to admit it. Perhaps this is because it reminds us too much of our mortality.

Kohut believed that to develop self structure and coherence we need self-selfobject relationships. He says we need them to nourish us to gain coherence. He says that selfobjects are as important to us as a limb of our bodies or the oxygen we breathe. Kohut tells that we metabolize our mothers and other selfobjects like a kind of protein, and that through this act over time, we build self-structure.

What is remarkable about Kohut's language is that it is a language of body acting as the language of psyche. It is a symbolic language that is as physical as it is because Kohut, I think, wants to give us a bodily sense of the power of words, words that actually have the ability to transform and change the psyche/soma – mind/body as a unit. This is what I have implied throughout this book when I use the words "liminal," and "imaginal."

Liminal describes a state of being on the threshold between and within both body and mind, and imaginal expresses the substantial quality of images to transform us physically as well as mentally. Images are substantial in that they have the power to build self-structure. They are transformative. Indeed, they are what some mean by "transubstantiation." They bring us from our physical bodies into a realm of relationship with the divinities, as Heidegger says. They bring us to a space of transcendence, understanding that we are more than physical beings, and less than immortal beings (who have nothing but ambrosia running through their veins). All this we achieve through the miracle of language, the substance of words that live in the double-entendres of symbol, metaphor, and meaning that makes us into what we know to be human. We live and play in paradox. It is not a far step from this to understanding the mystical, extraordinary world that we are always aware of, and long to pin down conceptually, but never can. This world is what C.G. Jung calls the "psychoid," the Sufis, "subtle body," Greeks, "demigods," and Christians "angels," and the Word, or Jesus, embodying both mortal and divine worlds. This is the nature of self, although we may never fully know it, because we are who we are, living always, as Kohut says, with a sense of melancholy as tragic rather than guilty selves, and with a sense of melancholy because we are creatures of transience.

But mourning, especially in more recent emphases on connecting with our dead substantially in more poetic and integrative ways and by looking anthropologically at the burial customs and beliefs of cultures other than our own, can bring us closer to the fuller world of interconnectedness with the extraordinary that we seek as part of who we are – closer to the liminal and imaginal fields some of us, like myself, yearn for.

I refer back to the dream I had of my mother drowning and then rising up again as Dr. Wolf. This was no wish-fulfillment dream but, rather, a dream of expressing other realms of possibility of metamorphic change that I know very little about, except that it builds self-structure, and the certainty of knowledge that I am who I am – that I have a self, built through the microprocesses of transmuting internalization. Everything flows, changes, and shares substance in myriads of different interrelated ways; we are always both one and many. That is how we carry our past and future with us. And it is in greeting and staying in relationships that we (and they) can go on growing and developing.

During the time I was with Dr. Wolf, I also sought out authors who wrote about the phenomenon of holding on to grieving after Freud's great work on Mourning and Melancholia, recognizing that although I had a strong sense that Freud was correct in what he said, it didn't do me much transformative good.

It was during this time that I came across the writings of George Hagman (2001, 2016), who amplifies and qualitatively changes Freud's language of cathexis and decathexis, by finding descriptive and powerful ways to integrate the dead and to take them with us as we move into the future.

Hagman (2001, 2016), shows us that there is a major paradigm shift from understanding the necessity to de-cathect the lost object to finding ways to transform it and integrate it with ourselves:

> Mourning refers to a varied and diverse psychological response to the loss of an important other. Mourning involves the transformation of the meaning and affects associated with one's relationship to the lost person, the goal of which is to permit one's survival without the other while at the same time insuring a continuing experience of relationship with the deceased. … An important aspect of mourning is that experience of disruption in self organization due to the loss of the function of the relationship with the other in sustaining self experience. Thus, mourning involves a reorganization of the survivor's sense of self as a key function of the process.
> (2001, p. 5)

Hagman resonates with my analysis in a deeply mirroring and affirming way. Dr. Wolf engaged my own sense of self disruption and fragmentation due to the traumatic loss of my mother by not only helping me to transform my self experience, but to recuperate self parts (that is, the selfobject functions that my mother had performed as well as those that she was also unable to perform), by creating an experience of a "continuing relationship with the deceased." Dr. Wolf did this by sharing his "protein" with me in such a way that in my own dream life he actually became my mother. The power of the dream was substantial enough to bring her to life for me with a certainty that was fully emotionally healing.

Greg Mogenson's work, *Greeting the Angels* (1992) adds a poetic and Jungian sensibility to the way the self reorganizes in mourning due to the loss of the relationship with the other. While close to George Hagman's ideas, Mogenson's more poetic, depth perspective on mourning provided a way for me to fall into an imaginal, ritual space where I came to sense a shared embodiment with my mother:

> The absent object, precisely by virtue of being absent, is no longer what we see but how we see.[1] Perception is a nostalgic

> phenomenon; there is a longing in it, a longing which causes us to see what's "out there" in terms of what is no longer "out there" at all.
>
> (1992, p. 10)

What Mogenson tells us is that the mourning process, if it is not to focus simply on the encrusted corporeity of the human body, must grow through the imaginal, which is the authentic language of the psyche. We need not mourn the dead as dead but rather allow them to grow within our own imaginal worlds. It is the presence of their absence that becomes real within our psyches, which sloughs off the dead person in terms of how they are actually remembered. Once they begin to become alive again for us through the imaginal, they form within us as part of ourselves. The imaginal, then, is the substantive imagery of what Kohut calls the protein that we metabolize from our selfobjects to build self structure.

The beloved dead are not simply recuperated for the sake of helping us to recuperate, nor "decathected," as Freud says, nor "internalized." They turn up in our imaginations in a living relationship, and being alive, they grow alongside us. As we grow, we grow our ghosts. They transform from ghosts to ancestors. As imaginal, they re-flesh themselves to join a living culture of the imagination.

In my own understanding of what happened with Dr. Wolf, I felt that I was able to give up the personal mother that I so intimately struggled with and mourned in my short time with her – the mother who became so intimately and ambivalently tied up with my own transferences and projections. With Dr. Wolf as a catalyzing and transformative presence, she could now join with me, and I could feel us growing alongside and in one another. In the process our own ancestry came into consciousness, at least as far back as I could remember. So much that had previously been lost in shadow began to become clear and real, making it possible for me to bring it forward into the future.

Reading Hagman and Mogenson deepened my sense of having rediscovered a mother who could become my companion throughout life, bringing her own past with her. In the process, and perhaps most important, this experience also brought together my understandings of Jung and self psychology.

This coming together of the two deepest influences in my psychological life brought me back to Greeks, and the notion of immortality as a continuous cycling of generations. I felt myself moving deeply into a maternal idiom of cycling in a nature full of many gods:

> The meaning of birth is not the beginning of all things, not the unique, the original beginning but continuity in an uninterrupted sequence of births. In the identity of mother and daughter, the eternally child-bearing mother manifests herself as an eternal being.... The child is that sign that this duration is more than individual: that it is continuity and continual rebirth in one's own offspring.
>
> (Jung and Kerenyi, 1963, p. 162)

5.5 Incorporating the Greeks into a New Vision of Selfhood

I had earlier delighted in the similarity between the archaic psyche's connections with nature, community and the sacred (as expressed through Homeric narratives and archaic Greek literature) and the liminal, imaginal realms that I had experienced as my own reality as a child. I felt deeply affirmed by the thought that my experiences were reflected in the more openly acknowledged liminal reality of the archaic Greek world. Dr. Wolf had helped me to rediscover my mother and feel her as a companion as we grew together into a maturing self-selfobject relationship. The imaginal third spaces, as described further by Hagman and Mogenson, in which this new relationship was taking place, gave me a new sense of reality and safety.

I could now, after the analysis, feel that my mother was with me. The presence of her absence no longer had a haunting ghostlike quality, but warmth and a feeling of connectedness. This must be, I thought, how it felt to be in living touch with the gods. For the Greeks, the gods populated the human world, connecting it and all of nature with divinity. Jung might say of the gods, as he did of alchemical substances and the gold of the philosopher's stone, that they were mere projections of our inner experiences onto a cosmic landscape. I could not believe that. For me, the gods were individuals, alive and substantial. I felt that they communicated with me as they communicated with the ancient Greeks. Dr. Wolf, in his metamorphosis as my mother, made both the gods and my mother idealized presences to count on, whether or not they were actually there. He healed my sense of isolation and confusion.

Once again, I find myself struggling with more common western notions that this was all just "imagination" and perhaps "poetizing" as a way to escape reality – perhaps, at its worst, even a psychotic way of thinking. I sensed something quite different, a perception of time and space as a sheer expanse of freedom and integration extending far beyond myself as a human being and into a new kind of "wholeness" (cf. Kulka, 2021).

The conversation between contemporary psychoanalysis and the archaic (rather than the classical) Greeks seems essential because both seek to come to terms with a psyche that has not yet established any sense of a coherent self-structure, but can be understood through connectedness with nature, community and the sacred. This sense of profound and often ineffable connectedness is what contemporary self and relational psychotherapies seek to establish between themselves and their patients.

The later Classical period, especially the world of Athens, sought to develop a new kind of individual that would be able to function more comfortably in the new civic state. These individuals needed to develop an autonomous interiority that led to their being more self-reliant and politically responsible. To do this, they were compelled to slough off and devalue much that had been essential in a now fading tribal and heroic world.

Perhaps the connection with a matrilineal world with its reverence for a great mother nature and seasonal cycles of birth and death threatened the budding patriarchy in its assertion of patrilineality. Previously, mothers alone could identify the sons of any particular father. The power of the Great Mother now showed herself as the face of a Medusa because she was too threatening for the individuating, budding, interior psyche that was just coming into being to feel comfortable with. She was omnipotent in that she gave birth to all beings but could destroy them at will. In her guise as Medusa, she was destructive, and petrifying because separating from her meant giving up the tribal world of a cyclical, seasonal and eternally repetitive space and time. The city-state saw this view of immortality and its interconnectedness unendurably threatening to its privileging of individuated linear and mortal lives, but there was still a longing for it, a nostalgia for an earlier and simpler time.

Many feminists in the 1970s, researching deeply into the meaning and ways of the great goddess cultures argue that we westerners have lost our connection to the maternal and what it represents. Christopher Bollas (1987) speaks of how the maternal idiom itself is essential for our transformation into individual selves in community. I believe that if we are going to restore a sense of lost vitality, fluidity and connectedness to our sense of self as a culture and to achieve egalitarianism in our increasingly interdependent world we need to reconnect with that earlier world.

Relational psychoanalysts seek to overcome ego boundaries and the idea of an autonomous self to engage in empathic third fields, that is, into the liminal and intermediate emotional and relational fields that connect us as subjects. Trying to do this from the perspective of an already established sociopolitical notion of the contemporary western, patriarchal self left to us by the Classical Greeks, makes this exceptionally difficult.

However, I think that gaining a sense of the psyche that inhabited the preclassical, polytheistic, and tribal world is a powerful way for theorists and clinicians to deepen their own sense of a potentially new psyche that can move us into a more integrated future world with all its challenges of change. Archaic Greek literature lends literary and conceptual power to contemporary relational fields that can deepen and expand the possibilities for how to create an enriched psychological life.

Remembering the beauty of liminality in my early childhood, and then experiencing the traumatizing violence of my mother's death with its accompanying ambivalence of rage and love, I now imagine a new kind of psyche, one that I believe was too fragile to take shape in the Classical Greek world and is just coming of age in ours. This idea of a transformed self involves moving from the strength of our integration as western sociopolitical selves as conceived by the Classical Greeks to future selves actively interconnected with nature, human and divine. Here, a powerful maternal idiom can join and transform the established patriarchal, sociopolitical world. Perhaps this new, more integrated self can perceive and safely embrace the idea of ecosystems and interconnectedness, accepting the world of others in whatever shape or form they emerge.

In the chapters that follow, I describe in much greater detail my understanding of how the move from a ritual to an archaic and then to the classical world of the Greeks resonates with contemporary forms of psychoanalysis, showing the importance of understanding the Great Mother as a larger transpersonal sense of the maternal, whom we as a culture have grown away from to create a separate and overly self-conscious self.

To experience the kind of self that I am imagining in such a way as to live it and to allow it to influence and expand our own clinical and theoretical perspectives, I believe we need to immerse ourselves in the writings of Homeric as well as Classical Greek texts. These will make it possible for us to reflect on the changes that give birth to the more familiar world of the 5th century in Athens. I will argue that attending to the imaginal, the imaginary, and the transformative power of symbols in these texts will help us to feel more of a sense of cohesion in the face of our chaotic contemporary world.

Myths express the loss of wholeness and immortality that many of us feel. The Garden of Eden myth expresses the agony of separation from god's paradisial garden through the development of the human consciousness of good and evil. The myth of Orpheus, lyre singer and poet, expresses the desire for the return of Eurydice, his lost love. Orpheus creates songs on his lyre that make even Death weep and stones come alive. Orphic songs symbolize the power of art to reconnect to the fullness of a union with nature that we have lost. They touch us through nostalgia, which means in Greek, the painful desire to return home.

It is works of art such as these that bring us into a sense of primal unity again. They can lead us into feelings of transformation, integrity, and a sense of liminal third fields that connect us intersubjectively.

Insofar as relational and intersubjective psychoanalysts are aware of the power of the liminal to connect with other psyches through reverie, intuition and empathic immersion, we are living in what Bollas calls an aesthetic, maternal idiom that can itself stimulate faith and hope in interconnectedness. This faith in turn issues forth into the growth of ourselves as humans who can incorporate the diversity of life and, indeed, the certainty of death into our very beings.

This book then becomes a tribute to the contributions of contemporary psychoanalysts who have begun to see the value of liminal and relational spaces to create individuals who do not fear, or shame, or blame themselves or others. It is a tribute to the return of care and the maternal in our sociopolitical structures. It is ultimately a call to the idea of the sacred that, as Neumann and Bollas tell us, precedes the maternal, but is inevitably joined with it.

Note

1 I allude here to Edward Casey's statement: "The image is not *what* is present to awareness – this is the content proper – but *how* this content is presented" (4, p. 10).

E. Casey, Toward a phenomenology of the imagination, *Journal of the British Society of Phenomenology*, 5 (1974).

References

Bollas, C. (1987). *The Shadow of the Object: Psychoanalysis of the UnthoughtKnown.* New York: Columbia University Press.

Dobson, M.W.D-S. (1984, July). Unpublished Journal.

Dobson, M.W.D-S. (2007). Freud, Kohut, Sophocles: Did Oedipus do wrong? *International Journal of Self Psychology*, 2(1).
Dobson, M.W.D-S. (2020). Young Kohut and the ancient Greek satyr play *Psychoanalysis, Self and Context*, 15(1).
Freud, S. (1917). Mourning and melancholia. Vol. 14, p. 239 of *The Standard Edition of the Complete Works of Sigmund Freud.* (J. Strachey, trans). London: Hogarth Press, pp. 1953–1974.
Grotstein, J. (1997). Internal objects or chimerical monsters. *Journal of Analytical Psychology* 42: 45–80.
Hagman, G. (2001). Beyond decathexis: Towards a new psychoanalytic understanding and treatment of mourning. In R. Neimeyer (ed.), *Meaning Reconstruction and the Experience of Loss*. Washington DC: American Psychological Association, pp. 13–31.
Hagman, G. (2016). New mourning: A new psychoanalytic understanding and treatment of mourning. In G. Hagman (ed.), *New Models of Bereavement Theory and Treatment: New Mourning* (Ch. 12). London: Routledge.
Heidegger, M. (1971). Building, dwelling, thinking. In J. Hofstadter (trans.), *Poetry, Language, Thought*. New York: Harper Colophon, pp. 145–162.
Jung, C.G. and Kerenyi, C. (1963). *Essays on a Science of Mythology: The Myth of the Divine Child and the Mysteries of Eleusis* (1973). Princeton, NJ: Princeton University Press.
Kerenyi, C. (1967). *Eleusis: Archetypal Image of Mother and Daughter* (Ralph Manheim, trans.). Princeton, NJ: Princeton University Press. (Original work published in 1960.)
Kohut, H. and Wolf, E. (1978). The disorders of the self and their treatment: An outline. In A. Morrison (ed.), *Essential Papers on Narcissism*. New York: New York University Press, pp. 175–196.
Kulka, R. (2021). Self psychology: The ethics of oneness. *Psychoanalytic Review* 108: 141–153.
Lachman, F. (2008). *Transforming Narcissism: Reflections on Empathy, Humor, and Expectations* (Psychoanalytic Inquiry Book Series, Vol. 28). London: Analytic Press: Taylor and Francis Group.
Mogenson, G. (1992). *Greeting the Angels: An Imaginal View of the Mourning Process.* Amityville, NY: Baywood Publishing Company.
Ogden, T.H. (2001). *Conversations at the Frontier of Dreaming.* (Ch. 8, pp. 203–236). Northvale, NJ: Jason Aronson.
Ornstein, P.H. (1980). Self-psychology and the concept of health. In A. Goldberg (ed.), *Advances in Self Psychology.* New York: International Universities Press.

Segal, H. (1964). *Introduction to the Work of Melanie Klein.* New York: Basic Books.

Winnicott, D.W. (1965a). The development of the capacity for concern. In *The Maturational Processes and the Facilitating Environment: Studies in the Theory of Emotional Development.* New York: International Universities Press, pp. 73–81.

Winnicott, D.W. (1971a). Dreaming, fantasying and living. In *Playing and Reality* (pp. 26–38). London: Routledge.

Wolf, E.S. (1978). *Treating the Self: Elements of Clinical Self Psychology.* New York: Guilford Press.

Zabriskie, B. (1997). Thawing the "frozen accidents": The archetypal view in countertransference. *Journal of Analytical Psychology,* 42: 25–40.

Part II

Archaic Permeability and Psychic Transformation in Greek Epic Poetry and Tragedy

Chapter 6

The Archaic Greek Heroic Psyche

All things flow

Heraclitus

6.1 Introduction

Archaic Greek concepts of identity are organized in ways that fragment our own view of self-coherence. The self is conceived in terms of a multiple collective, where boundaries melt between human, natural, and divine. This notion of psyche mixes familiar categories of substantial and insubstantial, matter and psyche, visible and invisible. The archaic Greeks redraw (from our perspective) the circumference of self, to include an engagement and flow with the rest of the cosmos. Indeed, the Greek heroic vision might see our conception of ego as fragmented, rather than as bounded or centered, and as having broken away from its cosmic and cultural webs.

Rather than existing in a psychological, transitional space bounded by subject/fantasy on one side and object/reality on the other, the heroic world takes transitional space as primary atmosphere, as the space from which subject and object are created, rather than the other way around. The gods, monsters, even personified mental concepts and emotions that inhabit the Homeric world can in no way be considered "projections" of the human subject onto the screen of the cosmos, because the thinking, cohering, internalized subject does not yet exist. There is no alternate language in which to frame the undifferentiated,

DOI: 10.4324/9781003340751-8

irrational face of war, except as Ares, or to speak of eros, except as Aphrodite (cf. Snell, 1953/1960; Onians, 1951).

Although contemporary interpreters may be able to translate this world into a psychological internal-external frame of Kleinian object relations, of the archetypal world of Jung, or even into the more multiply imaged object worlds of Grotstein and Bollas, the world as the archaic Greeks experienced it did not have these languages. If we were to try to translate their perceptions into our formulations, we might say that the heroes lived in a cosmos that could be construed as open, expanded, space, with little sense of themselves as selves existing outside or beyond that space. They were neither merged in or fused with it, nor were they autonomous in our terms. Their sense of self-coherence actually included nature, human, and the sacred. It was a communal self, a tribal self, permeated by divinities and other forces that appeared to them to course through their beings, flowing inside, outside, and around them. Often Homeric heroes appeared to be more strongly connected in their various body parts to gods and other outside forces than those parts were to one another.

6.2 The Heroic Body

A given culture's idea of psyche cannot be well-formulated without understanding its view of the body. Thus, in order to understand more fully the difference between modern and heroic Greek self-concepts, we need to look at the way body is conceived: "The way in which we understand and treat our bodies is a reflection of the way in which we understand and treat the world" (Romanyshyn, 1992, p. 103).

In western culture, we tend to think of our bodies as coherent, working machines, quite closed from the outside except for the orifices. The modern body is "a body, finally, which has no contact with the surrounding atmosphere, a body closed in upon itself and insulated from the world" (Romanyshyn, p. 103). In contrast, when we attempt to determine the Greek notion of body, we find ourselves in a bewildering distribution of ancient

Greek terms that indicate a quite different body conception from the one we are used to.

The archaic Greeks lived in a world of sacrificial rituals and wars, where to view dead bodies of both men and animals were commonplace. Bodies were imminently corruptible. Yet, this did not give rise to a religious attitude that worshipped a disembodied psyche as the only form of permanence and goodness. Rather, the body itself was the object of worship in all its youth, prowess, beauty, and vitality. The *aristeia* of a warrior hero, that moment in which he was "the best and most noble," came at the height of battle, when he was exerting all the bodily strength he had against the enemy. At this moment of crisis, face to face with an opponent who might instantly take his life, the warrior participated in a supreme aliveness of living in the absolute moment. It was this that gave him the sense of feeling most gloriously and physically immortal. It was also in that moment that the hero possessed *arete*, translated as "virtue" in Plato's time. In Homer, virtue meant the height of one's manly powers (*arē* and *vir* both evoke "male," in Greek and Latin respectively). Even in classical times, when soul began to be defined, it was commonplace to believe that a beautiful soul could not reside in anything but a beautiful body. The body was considered the mirror of the soul.

Heroic bodies, so valued for their beauty, strength, and aliveness, were quite permeable. Not only were the six orifices avenues of communication between these bodies and the outside, but every organ in the body was connected with a god. *Splanchna*, "innards," received the "image-impress" of gods (Padel, 1992, p. 17). Theagenes of Rhegium, in the 6th century BCE, allegorized Homer in terms of entrails, suggesting that "Apollo represented the gall, Demeter the liver, Dionysos, the spleen," and so forth (p. 17). Gods are in innards. The connection between them is "fluid, ambiguous, mercurial, transformative, and divine" (p. 11).

Through the common Greek practice of consulting entrails, human beings could "hear the gods speak" (Padel, p. 17). Aeschylus' Prometheus says he taught human beings "to watch for the *splanchna*'s smoothness, and what color a gall vessel should be to please gods; and the liver lobe's dappling symmetry" (quoted in Padel, 1992, p. 17).

The future was read by examining vitals, especially the liver. Innards were left on altars to be burned for the gods. If they did not burn or were not consumed by other living things, in other words, if the cycles and connections with other parts of nature were broken, it suggested ritual or emotional pollution. Even as late as Sophocles' *Antigone*, which was produced at the height of what is known as the classical period in the 5th century BCE, Creon's crime of refusing to bury the dead is expressed by the birds' unwillingness to touch the sacrifices on the altars. When we think of the body organs as connecting with gods and nature in this way, we can begin to see the multiple webbing that held psyches together. Skin itself, the body envelope, loses much of its sense of boundary, for outside and inside are intimately connected.

The fluidity of the cosmos in this worldview led to a sense that the human being was more multiply connected than unified as a conscious self. "Words for equipment of consciousness have a pluralizing effect, like the 'many names' of gods who so often affect the innards ... From the start, multiplicity is a core condition of consciousness, as of religion, in Greek thought" (Padel, 1992, p. 18). Since emotions and organs frequently had the same name, it can be assumed that they were identical, with no sense of separation of physical from mental qualities. And insofar as these organs were also the seats of the gods, who thought, talked, and behaved in certain ways, we can assume that the heroic body contained multiple centers of consciousness, which were easily permeable to the outside.

The fact is that in the archaic Greek period "corporeity" still does not acknowledge a distinction between body and soul, nor does it establish a radical break between the natural and the supernatural. Man's corporality also includes organic realities, vital forces, psychic activities, divine inspirations, or influxes. The same word can refer to each of these various domains. On the other hand, there is no term that designates the body as an organic unity that supports the individual in the multiplicity of his vital and mental functions. The word *soma*, translated as body, originally designated only a corpse (Vernant, 1991c, p. 30).

As long as the body is alive and inhabited by energy, it is expressed multiply, in terms such as *guia*, "supple body members," or *melea*, "limbs that hold force" (p. 30). Emotions, as well as the ability to know, may exist within the individual organic body, but they are equally flowing through that divine atmosphere in which it participates. In Vernant's view, the hero's "organic consciousness" senses "joy," "irritation," or "boldness," but they are breathed into him by a god:

> *Menas,* vital ardor, *alkē,* fortitude, *kratos,* the power of domination, *phobos,* fear, *eros*, the impetus of desire, and *lussa,* the warrior's frenzy, are all localized in the body, bound to the body they invest; but as "powers," these exceed and surpass every individual carnal shell. They can abandon it just as they invaded it. In the same way, when a man's spirit is blinded or enlightened, it is most often because, in the intimate recesses of his *nous* or his *phrenes,* a god intervenes to inspire the aberration of error, *atē,* or its contrary, a wise resolve.
>
> (Vernant, 1991c, p. 37)

Permeability is not simply metaphorical. Emotions and organs both appear to have physical properties that are liquid, that can actually flow or be breathed in and out of the body. *Cholos*, the Greek word for what the medievalists understood as the choleric humor, "seizes you, sinks into you, conquers you. You nurse, ripen, or quench it … it can be roused, be moved, boil over" (Padel, 1992, p. 24).

> *Nous*, the Greek word for "mind" or "intelligence," and one of the key words that might indicate an interior sense of "ego," or "I-ness" to a Cartesian, is what the ancient philosopher, Diogenes, called "air": All people are steered by it; it has power over everything. We smell with the "air around the brain."
>
> (Vernant, p.40)

The word *poras* became popular in the 4th century as a scientific term explaining how earlier Greeks understood the interaction between their bodies and the cosmos. *Poroi* are "pores," ways into and out of the body, in other words, channels and veins (p. 41). It is through the *poroi* that emotions, forces, and divine influences come. *Splanchna*, "innards," were thought by Aristotle in the 4th century to be situated on the "veiny *poroi*," and "like mud from a running stream" to be deposited by the ooze of blood through veins (p. 43). What is key here is that the whole cosmos is made of the same liquid stuff. "Body and mind" as well are made "of the same stuff as the world outside" (p. 43). Because of these connections, if the gods were in conflict, especially given that each god favored an organ of the human body, the hero himself felt disunified and torn apart. "Divinity, too, manifests 'unity through multiplicity,' and through its own self-conflict brings about self-conflicting damage in human innards" (p. 48).

The hero's body, while its permeability allows forces to pass through it, also extends in space and identity to its accoutrements. When Achilles, after he has given his own armor to his beloved Patroclus to go fight in his place near the Trojan Walls, dons the new armor fashioned for him by the god Hephaestus. His warrior's "vital ardor" or *menos* shines not only in his eyes, but in the brilliant bronze leaping in fire through the helmet's crest to the sky (cf. Homer, trans. R. Fagles, 1990). His *menos* is both given to him by the gods through the armor and shines back upon the cosmos. At this moment, Achilles becomes more than a man; he becomes his armor, and his armor becomes an extension of his body:

> And brilliant Achilleus tried himself in his armor, to see if it fitted close, and how his glorious limbs ran within it, and the armor became as wings and upheld the shepherd of the people.
>
> (Vernant, 1991c, p. 38 [*Iliad*, Bk. 19, ll 384–386])

Likewise, as Achilles becomes more than human through the donning of armor that is divine, his friend Patroclus is killed in Achilles' mortal armor, thereby indicating the death of the mortal Achilles. When personalities can be exchanged through armor, then the personality cannot be defined in terms of the modern self as we imagine it to be.

Appurtenances as well, like the scepter that Agamemnon inherited from his ancestors, are not merely signs and symbols of power; they are efficacious; they are links to a hero's inner energy. Agamemnon's scepter helps him to rule the army, but the very same scepter, in Achilles' hands, turns into a piece of dead wood, divested of its leaves and branches, never to grow again, recalling for us the often-quoted Homeric phrase, "as are the generations of leaves, so are the lives of mortal men" (Homer, 1990, trans. R. Fagles [*Il.* Bk.6., 1.171]), the scepter acquires the fate of Achilles and transforms as soon as it is given to him – the nature hero with the divine mother and little heritage, who will die young. Such appurtenances are equivalent to a person's limbs, and "together with the other parts of the body, define that person's bodily configuration" (Vernant, 1991c, p. 38).

In this worldview, objects themselves change and acquire the characteristics of what they are close to, in the same way that what they are close to or bound with can acquire their characteristics and take in their energy.

Heroes themselves transform in their very appearance by being affected from the outside. Grace and power can be poured upon them by a god. They can change their ages, and sometimes even disappear. Odysseus, washed up on the shores of Phaeacia, swollen and bruised by the sea, washes himself and is "made taller and more massive by Athena. with his hair curling down over his forehead" (Vernant. 1991c, p. 39. [Od. 6, 227–237]). Odysseus cleansing makes him more than he is to the onlooker. Athena can also turn Odysseus into a beggar, "bald and bleary eyed" (p. 39 [Od. 13. 429–435]), unrecognizable to his own wife and son, and then back again into a handsome youth, the way he was when he left Penelope 20 years earlier (Vernant, 1991c, p. 39). In the *Iliad*, when Aphrodite wishes to save the life of Paris (Vernant, p. 42 [Il.3. 373–382]), she whisks him off the battlefield in a mist, so making him invisible and astonishing those warriors on the verge of killing him who cannot understand where he has gone.

6.3 Gods and Heroes as Individuals?

In similar fashion, the gods themselves change and, in so doing, break down the categories which make us feel secure in our perceptions. Paradoxically, they can seem at the very same time both near and far, familiar and unfamiliar, heavy and light, visible to one person and invisible to all those around him. When Achilles is about to draw his sword on Agamemnon, Athena flies down to catch him by the hair. He recognizes her instantly; no one else sees her (Homer, trans. R. Fagles, 1990). When Poseidon appears as Calchas, the seer, to give confidence to the two Ajaxes, Ajax knows immediately that it is Poseidon by his feet and legs as he is disappearing:

Poseidon imitates the heavy gait of the old prophet, yet his step was like "a quick winged falcon pursuing a bird across the plain" (Vernant, 1991c, p. 43 [Il. 13. ll. 62–65]).

The divine body, in all the concentrated mass of its being, weighs as much as the marble or bronze statue located in the god's temple: yet it is aerial, ethereal, impalpable, and as weightless as a ray of light (p. 43).

Readers of the *Iliad* and the *Odyssey* might well object that for all that has been said about the permeability and changeability of the bodies of gods and heroes, and about the flow of the cosmos in which they all participate, they still appear quite individual. They still look, to all accounts and purposes, as if they had distinct selves and self-consciousness. Odysseus will never turn into Achilles. Athena will never become Aphrodite or Artemis.

If we consider that the way in which gods are conceived in a culture is a touchstone for understanding how a culture conceives itself, then we can say that particular personifications of the Greek gods indicate that there is indeed an increasing sense of differentiation among personalities in the heroic period than in earlier times and certainly than in other cultures.

To begin with, the Greek gods are humans, not animals. They are not snakes or elephants or turtles, or even partly so. In this way, Greek gods were always different from the gods of India or Egypt. From very early, they were humanized, and appear to have had quite specific functions. A look, for example, at Minoan art and its predecessors details a progression from three female goddesses divided into locations of hearth, harvest, and the wild, who were later to be named and more specifically characterized as Athena, Demeter, and Artemis. Athena is an outgrowth of a Minoan snake goddess who appears to rule the hearth. Depictions of this snake goddess show her with a snake twined around her waist. Athena, her successor, goddess of battle, and later of the city-state (the civic home), is also associated with a snake, but in sculpture, it curls inside her shield and rests on her aegis as the snaky head of Medusa. Neither goddess ever actually appears as a snake, but both probably go back to an earlier Near Eastern goddess who combined the powers of governance, battle, and eros as well.

In the heroic world, Athena gains family, appearing as a favored daughter of Zeus. She shares her father's wisdom and drives a war chariot. She could not be confused with Aphrodite, the tender and emotional goddess of beauty, or Hera, the wily wife of Zeus. However, if we look more closely, we can see that although these immortals have names and characteristics, they are not yet distinct personalities. Rather, they are cultural stereotypes, embodying functions as well as universals.

Already, this begins to break down another of our cherished categories for making sense of the world. In embodying specific functions and universals, the gods are at the same time specific and universal. The contemporary thinker, trained in the division between body and soul, and understanding that the particular cannot be universal, may find it hard to comprehend how the gods can participate in universal categories while having specific characteristics. Yet where we would see fragmentariness and distinctiveness as inevitably limiting, the archaic Greeks, especially as represented in the writings of Hesiod, see the characteristics of the gods as defining specific functions and universals that balance together in an eternal and unshakeable order: "If the gods possess plenitude, perfection, immutability, it is because at the end of the process that led to the emergence of a stable, organized and harmonious cosmos, each divine person's individuality is clearly fixed" (Vernant, 1991c, p. 48). Thus, the very particularity of a god is what gives that god its "universal inexhaustible power" (p. 48).

In other words, although the gods appear to be particular, they are in fact representing together a harmony of functions and universals. This harmony constitutes a unity, but it is a unity of multiples. This appears as yet one more expression of the multiply cohering psyche. To make the matter yet more complex, as worshipped in cult, each god has many different and anomalous functions. Even when they appear singular and distinct on the large canvas of heroic narrative, they are also, as understood by the common culture, too multiple in their various functions to be considered fully coherent. Zeus, for example, can be called upon in his functions of weather god, or as the god of hospitality, or of the underworld, and so forth (cf. Farnell, 1896–1909; Burkert, 1985). Another basic determinant of individual identity is location. Although each god appears to have a domain, for example Poseidon rules the sea, Zeus the heavens, and Pluto the deep underworld, to expect to find a god in his or her location only is somewhat short-sighted. Gods appear to be able to change appearance and body at will, and to take on the guise of an Homeric warrior at the same time that they are pervasive in their own domain.

Gods are also immortal, which means that they have no age and no mortality. If body determines specific location, and time a certain chronological progression through life, then the gods partake in neither: "In a single impulse, the gods' corporeal vitality extends across past, present, and future, in the same way that its energy is deployed to the ends of the universe" (Vernant, 1991c, p. 46).

But what of the hero? Does he not have a name and a location as well as particular characteristics that are fixed in time and space? Does not the very heroic emphasis on body reinforce his individuality, his personal identity, his capacity for agency? In fact, the hero is an individual and agent only in the context of his tribe, and through a complex network of communal values. Even his relationship with the divine is established through the community. Impiety, *asebeia*, wronging the gods, is equivalent to wronging one's community (Vernant, 1983a, p. 326). Indeed, the example of Hippolytus in Euripides' tragedy of the same name, who dedicated himself only to Artemis, shows that devotion to one god alone, which might begin to determine a particular personality structure, could lead to annihilation (cf. Caldwell, 1985; Devereux, 1985). It was important to honor all the gods – in other words, to be aware of and to embody multiple characteristics. A look at 6th- and 5th-century Greek statuary of young men, *kouroi*, only confirms the sense that there is no individualization; rather, the statues all are formed to represent the universalizing ideals of strength, grace, and beauty.

Personal identity, it might be argued, is also based on the sense that persons have of their own integrated center – their soul, their intelligence, or as we might say in contemporary psychology, their ego – a sense of personal agency distinct and separate from those of others. But, once again, these words for possible integrity and wholeness have quite different and less integrative senses in the archaic Greek world.

That which we might want to call the hero's soul, the translation of the Greek word *psyche*, drifts around outside and inside him. Heroes do not have psyches, in our sense of the term. Psyche, a word connected to breath, is only used as a term after someone has died. It is a phantom that bears the same shape and appearance as the deceased hero, but it lacks a real existence (Vemant, 1991d, p. 187). It is not mentioned as providing coherence in life, and drifts as a fleshless replica of the body after death. *Nous*, the word for "intelligence," has already been mentioned as connected with air. It is a word that originally comes from an Indo-European root "*ne," which means "return to light and life." The Greek verb *neomai*, which comes from this root as well, means to "sail," or "to return" (Nagy, 1990, p. 218). *Nostos*, another derivative of *neomai* means "homecoming" (p. 218).

Homer's *Odyssey* is a favorite text in the western world because of its depiction of the making of a hero whose wily, many-turning intelligence outwits the forces of nature and the gods to return home (both from Troy, and from Hades, the world of death). In this text, it is clear that "the return home," *nostos*, by sailing across the sea, *neomai*, is dependent on Odysseus' *nous*, "intelligence" (Nagy, 1990, p. 219, and cf. Frame, 1978). What this suggests is that "intelligence" is connected with being able to return home, that is, to light and life, or to consciousness, rather than to the forgetfulness (*lethe*) of death. So *nous*, in the *Odyssey*, is perhaps in the linguistic process of coming to mean our inner home, the center of our intelligence, as well as that which allows us to navigate – to have and to execute our intentions. But, in the *Iliad* especially, and even in the *Odyssey*, we are still only on the verge of this capacity. *Nous* appears at best to be an easily swayed and all too quickly lost capacity for navigation in a permeable cosmos.

6.4 Heroic Stability

A contemporary psychologist of self might wonder whether the Homeric hero could rest at all comfortably in such permeability. Was there no quest at all for permanence or stability in this world of psychic multiplicity, where there was no boundedness of the individual self and no sense of any eternal afterlife?

Homeric heroes sensed deeply their own mortality in an environment in which there was no belief in an eternal soul. Despite this, the very ways in which they celebrated permanence brought a greater stability to their lives than we can imagine, given their understanding of the inter-webbing of all material and nonmaterial beings. This stability was achieved through the confidence of the heroes that they would be memorialized, and in this way would achieve everlasting fame.

Homeric society put great emphasis on memorializing their heroes. The memory of the hero is preserved by recounting tales of his glory. *Kleos*, however, which might be thought of as the remembered glory of the hero in narrative, is more substantial than we might think. The memory in fame of a hero is not just a remembered story that brings that hero back to life in the telling through a kind of reminiscing. Just as bodies are more permeable than we consider them to be, so are words more substantial. Words have power. They can move into and through their hearers like gods, effecting transformations and bringing the hero into virtual reality, as the hearers feel themselves to intermingle with the heroes and to share alike in their substance and fame. This perhaps lends a greater sense of permanence to narrative and memory than we might accord them.

Part of the reason for the presence and power of words in recollection is that Homeric poetry was created orally by a number of poets over a long period of time (cf. Stolz and Shannon, 1976). The poems, therefore, become poems in the process of their being told and in the context in which they were told. Homer's *Iliad* was always performed. It was not first written. What this means is that it does not exist outside of memory and without the "mind-act" of remembering (Bakker, 1997, p. 15). Time coalesces in the act of re-membering, yet another form of the melting of categories of distinction. The past, in fact, becomes present, both in a temporal and in a spatial sense: It is turned from "then" and "there" into "now" and "here" within the context of a special social event and throughout the actions of a special, authoritative speaker. "Epic discourse strives to overcome the gap between the natural, visual icon and the arbitrary sign that is language, producing a sustained attempt at *enargeia* (vividness). It brings the far together with the near in both time and space" (p. 15).

Bakker defines this state of consciousness as "pretended immediacy" (1997, p. 15). The poet speaks the epic events of the past as if actually seeing them in the present. Very much like a modern-day storyteller, the poet thus engages the participation of the audience, who also, like children, feel themselves living the past in the immediacy of the present.

Winnicott describes "transitional space" as collapsing our sense of time into a continuous present that engages spontaneity and creative activity as the child feels the simultaneity of the creating moment with that which was already there and lives the middle space of the engagement of the two. In the same way, oral poetry brings its heroes and their past to its audience as moments of re-creation that feel like original creation, thus lending them a sense of authenticity and home.

For the oral poet and his audience, *aletheia*, "the absence of forgetfulness," creates the closest experience to the experience of truth as authenticity that one can imagine, because it is not simply the retelling of a story, but the affective creation of a narrative emerging from a collective oral tradition that is felt by its audience as an embodied home.

In linguistic studies of the ancient languages, particularly in the comparison of ancient Greek with Sanskrit and Avestan, we can see that even words themselves melt boundaries between the natural, mortal, and divine worlds and, in so doing, create a sense of subtle body that holds psyche together with the cosmos.

If we examine words such as "thunder," "dew," or "fire," we can see that all of them, while seemingly held within given constructs of gods and social beliefs, quickly rejoin, in the way their etymological patterns show themselves, other parts of the cosmos (Boedeker, 1984). This, in itself, while denying the potential sense of power for us in the separateness of language from the cosmos, gives people who hold to this worldview a sense of permanence by virtue of finding that words themselves participate in the material of creation.

When we look, for example, at the etymologies of the two major words for "dew," we not only see that they are used in contexts of fertility, but that this fertility connects sky, earth, animals, and human beings. In addition, they become a basic and generative image/substance for poetic speech and, among other things, the rule of kings. Boedeker calls this "the archaeology of an image" (1984, p. 6), whose beginnings and consequent development show us that the image remains as substance even as it takes on the conceptual weight of cultural and political framings in narrative. Thus the substance of dew becomes the substance of speech, and the word is not left as a concept removed from the material of its creation. In fact, it is the very substance of the image, in this case, "dew," that permeates and thereby joins seemingly disparate themes and structures. "Analogies of dew assimilate language to the realm of physical nature" (Boedeker, 1984, p. 98; cf. Detienne, 1996, p. 55).

In terms of its relationship to other liquids, a closer look at the word "dew" shows relationships that reveal conceptual and mythical connections. The words *eerse* and *drosos* signify dew in ancient Greek and are related. *Eerse* is a thematic noun from the root *wers-*; it is cognate with Indic *varsam* "rain," and Hittite *warsas*, "dew" and is related to Irish *frass* "rain" (Boedeker, 1984, p. 2). In ancient Greek, it is also related to the word for the sky god, Ouranos, as well as the verb *oureo,* to "urinate." The root *wers* also produces derivatives meaning "male animal": India *ursa-bha*, "bull, male," Latin *verres*, "boar," as well as the Latin *ros,* which means "dew," or "pure water." Through these etymologies, we can understand a context in which urine can be confused with semen, and males through generative dew appear to be the fecundators of the cosmos (p. 4). Further, we can see that through the word "dew," as Boedeker says, "the natural world coalesces with the divine on one hand and the human on the other, sometimes providing a very direct medium through which the two may communicate with each other" (p. 9).

In the Hymn to the Kouretes, a 4th century BCE text from Crete that clearly refers to a much earlier ritual, Zeus is hailed as "Lord of all that is wet and gleaming" (Harrison, 1962b, p. 7). The word for "wet and gleaming," *ganos*, has a number of different dictionary meanings, ranging from all that is wet and fertile, to all that is shimmering and brilliant (p. 9). In this Hymn, which calls for the earth to spring up crops, the flocks to reproduce, and the city itself to be prosperous, we see the essence of reproductivity and burgeoning to be in the liquids of the cosmos.

When we consider what is "wet and gleaming," we imagine dew and rain as well as all the liquids of birth and reproduction: semen, milk, vaginal fluids, and blood itself. Honey as well is a transforming liquid for the ancient Greeks and other cultures, as it comes from bees who produce it seemingly from the dew of the flower and make it into a substance that nurtures as well as preserving the body after death.

The Cretan Zeus, who is being honored and who is in fact present among his worshippers in this Hymn, is none other than Dionysus, the polymorphous god, who through his self-sacrifice, fragmentation, and reintegration into the bodies of his believers as they perform the rites of *sparagmos* (the tearing apart and eating of raw flesh) allows the regeneration of the earth's substances every year (Harrison, 1962b, p. 30). So do liquids become body and form beliefs and rituals, words serving as the material substance that allows transformation to occur. If memory, stone, and word all participate in material as well as immaterial qualities, then they are not objectively separate for the archaic Greeks as they are for us. They are caught up in a world of mutual participation. This suggests that in permeability itself there may be permanence and a sense of cosmic home.

References

Bakker, E. (1997). Storytelling in the future: Truth, time and tense in Homeric epic. In E. Bakker and A. Kahane, *Written Voices, Spoken Signs: Tradition, Performance, and the Epic*. Cambridge, MA: Harvard University Press, pp. 11–37.

Boedeker, D. (1984). *Descent from Heaven: Images of Dew in Greek Poetry and Religion.* Chico, CA: Scholar Press.

Burkert, W. (1985). *Greek Religion.* London: Basil Blackwell.

Caldwell, R. (1985). The power of Aphrodite: Eros and the boundaries of the self in the *Hippolytus.* In P. Burian (ed.), *Directions in Euripidean Criticism.* Durham, NC: Duke University Press, pp. 52–110.

Detienne, M. (1996). *The Masters of Truth in Archaic Greece* (J. Lloyd, trans.). New York: Urzone.

Devereux, G. (1985). *The Character of the Euripidean Hippolytos: An Ethno-psychoanalytical Study.* Chico, CA: Scholar Press.

Farnell, L.R. (1896–1909). *The Cults of the Greek states* (Vols. I–V). London: Oxford University Press.

Frame, D. (1978). *The Myth of Return in Early Greek Epic*. New Haven, CT: Yale University Press.

Harrison, J.E. (1962b). *Themis: A Study of the Social Origins of Greek Religion*. Cleveland: Meridian Press.

Homer (1990). *The Iliad* (Robert Fagles, trans.). New York: Viking Penguin.

Nagy, G. (1990). *Greek Mythology and Poetics*. Ithaca, NY: Cornell University Press.

Onians, R.B. (1951). *The Origins of European Thought* (2nd ed.). Cambridge, UK: Cambridge University Press.

Padel, R. (1992). *In and Out of the Greek Mind: Greek Images of the Tragic Self*. Princeton, NJ: Princeton University Press.

Romanyshyn, R. (1992). *Technology as Symptom and Dream*. Routledge: London.

Snell, B. (1960). *The Discovery of the Mind* (T.G. Rosenmeyer, trans.). Oxford: Oxford University Press. (Original work published 1953.)

Stolz, B.A. and R.S. Shannon (eds.) (1976). *Oral Literature and the Formula*. Ann Arbor, MI: University of Michigan Press.

Vernant, J.P. (1983a). Personal identity and religion. In *Myth and Thought Among the Greeks*. London: Routledge & Kegan Paul, pp. 321–341.

Vernant, J.P. (1991c). Mortals and immortals: The body of the divine. In F.I. Zeitlin (ed.), *Mortals and Immortals: Collected Essays*. Princeton, NJ: Princeton University Press, pp. 27–49.

Vernant, J.P. (1991d). *Psuche:* Simulacrum of the body or image of the divine? In F.I. Zeitlin (ed.), *Mortals and Immortals: Collected Essays*. Princeton, NJ: Princeton University Press, pp. 186–194.

Chapter 7

The Heroic Psyche

A Model for a Contemporary Self?

Heroic psyches lived and died in a battlefield of violent play. Everything about their world, especially in the *Iliad*, screamed out their ambivalence between desiring to stay in a horrendously bloody and fragmenting conflict over who was to possess Helen of Troy, on the one hand, and the desire to give up the war, go home, and farm in peace, on the other. Both sides of this ambivalence appear to have as their driving motive the possession of an archetypal feminine, either as the ideal beauty, Helen, or a ritual life lived out peaceably in seasonal agricultural cycles, which are usually connected with matricentrism.

One could hypothesize that the savage battles between the Trojans and Greeks themselves were symbolic of the intensity of the conflict between these two worlds: one, Troy, that was matricentric and peacefully oriented, the other, Greek, patriarchal and conflict driven, where women were required as possessions to validate patrilineal bloodlines.

The savage rage that the major heroic figures Achilles and Agamemnon exhibit against each other over the theft of women – a rage that seems to radiate to the very edges of the Homeric cosmos – suggests that this was indeed a traumatic period in ancient Greek culture. The combination of instability and rage, particularly when the rage has to do with the theft of women, in and of itself shows women's crucial importance both in their presence and absence throughout this transitional period.

The *Iliad* begins with Achilles' wrath over Agamemnon's theft of his prize woman, Briseis. Agamemnon demands Briseis as his own recompense for the loss of his prize woman Chryseis, whom

DOI: 10.4324/9781003340751-9

he is compelled to return to her priest father in order to save the Greek army from plague. The entire Trojan war was fought over the loss of Helen, the wife of Menelaus, whom Paris stole and took to Troy and over whom the Greeks originally went to war. It is usually stated that women were the most valued objects of stolen booty, better even than gold. They classified the hierarchical power of the Greek tribes – who came first, who was best, who had most honor. But why are women so important? The material is highly suggestive.

The combination of instability and rage felt by the Greek heroes over the loss and theft of their women is eerily like the dynamics theorized by Klein, Winnicott, Neumann, and others as occurring during the transitional phase of infant development. Winnicott's baby is supremely permeable because it as yet has nothing approaching self-coherence. In its helplessness and uncertainty of agency, it is constantly bursting forth with rage when it does not receive appropriate maternal nourishment. It struggles similarly when faced with its own ambivalence of wanting to be independent of its mother, but simultaneously needing her for help in developing its own capacities.

The world is dangerous enough in the presence of a good-enough mother, but in the presence of a traumatizing or absent mother, the world is devastating. For all its joys of oceanic bliss, immersion, and permeability in the sense of a maternal surround, the infant world can all too easily turn into a fearfully dangerous place when the maternal is physically or psychologically absent when needed. The only possible responses to this are rage or psychic deadness (cf. Eigen, 1996). The Homeric heroes chose rage.

7.1 The Psychological Development of Culture

To compare the transitional period of the Trojan War with the transitional experience of infant development, we need to imagine the Trojan War as involving a movement away from the mother, as well as to envision the psychic space of the hero as a developmental moment in a culture where the notion of self-consciousness was just beginning to emerge. In order to do this, we need to posit an analogous stage previous to the heroic world which felt itself merged with a matricentric tribal culture, which then births itself somewhat violently into a transitional and ambivalent space of gods and battles, then finally begins to attain "self-mastery" and becomes "one man instead of many, self-controlled and in unison" (Plato, 1961, eds. Hamilton and Cairns, *Rep*. 443e).

A number of psychologically and social-minded classical scholars have understood the development of ancient Greek culture in such a way as to validate the above line of argument (cf. Snell, 1960; Harrison 1962a; Neumann, 1973; Jaynes, 1976). To follow their developmental view of a person and culture and try to extend it to the psyche we have just been exploring, we have to accept that for all its beauty of permeability, the heroic psyche was chaotic and conflicted for the heroes themselves, who felt overly vulnerable and ultimately in too much conflict to survive. In this view, the heroic psyche becomes only an intermediate stage to the attainment of a coherent internalized self, which is regarded without question by Socrates and Plato as an ultimate goal. Plato argues, and the contemporary psychologist might agree, that one cannot one live when one feels oneself vulnerable enough to be killed if one looks a god in the face, or when one comes into conflict with one's own inner centers whenever the gods argue. If every god has a different provenance, then, as Socrates argues in the *Euthyphro*, how can one be pious to them all?

Seen in the above light, for all the joys and polytheistic pleasures of the heroic world, the heroic psyche cannot stand in any conceivable way as a comfortable model for a healthy, multiple, interdependent self. Nevertheless, reading through the spirited imagination of Homer's *Iliad*, which celebrates the very extremes of the heroes' ability to survive and thrive in the heights of rage, may stretch our own modern psychic structures, giving us permission to be ebullient, open, and free in a less constrained and ego-isolated atmosphere. The vibrant sense of psychic permeability and acceptance of multiplicity in connection with nature and the sacred can serve as a model for our own opening into third fields and potential interconnectedness. Yet, the line of development this sense took in Classical Greek culture, in which such flow and connection with natural forces was gradually negated, brought it into a false and highly fragile sense of autonomy. We, as westerners, have inherited this fragile, psychic structure as well, and use it all too unconsciously as a paradigm for the healthy self in contemporary western culture.

One could justify and explain the Trojan war by citing the breaking of important communal laws of guest friendship and reciprocity, or taking the rational view of the classical historian Thucydides (1951) that the necessity of retrieving women is simply an elaborate and ornamental fiction for the more mercenary motive of piracy. Many scholars do. But fiction, or myth, is what shows to us the actual psychic states of a population. Myth is cultural belief.

Simply and starkly expressed, as it is in the *Iliad*, what brings about the rage that devastates two populations is the presence and absence of women. This rage might well have to do with the fact that the *Iliad* was composed over the course of several centuries, during which there was an increasing recognition of the loss of a tight, tribal, and familial world that centered on the female, a world that was matrilineal and matricentric, if not matriarchal. If we look more closely at the *Iliad* now with this view in mind, we can see that it begins with rage and ends with death and deep social fragmentation. What came before this rage? Was there an earlier matricentric tribal world? One that could act and engage communally with the gods and with nature without conflict?

7.1.1 Jane Ellen Harrison

Jane Ellen Harrison, an all-too-easily-dismissed but recently retrieved author, whose work is increasingly cited by feminist and depth psychologists, gives evidence that such a world might have occurred (1962a, 1962b). Harrison was a classicist and an art historian who first had the audacity to suggest that studying ancient art might yield an understanding, mute as it was, of the origins of Greek belief. She followed in the footsteps of the great Cambridge anthropologists and classicists, Sir James Frazer (*The Golden Bough*, 1911–15). Gilbert Murray (*Five Stages of Greek Religion*, 1955), and Frances Cornford (*From Religion to Philosophy*, 1912). Harrison studied the 19th-century anthropologists, Emile Durkheim, Marcelle Mauss, and Levy-Bruhl. Her thesis was powerful, and although written in the throes of recent Darwinian theory, is in many respects still highly provocative and convincing today.

Harrison suggests that the earliest rituals for which we have record are the rituals that celebrate the seasons. These rituals, of a hunter-gatherer and then agricultural world, have as their focus the celebrations of a Great Mother Earth, who is all powerful in birth and death. She gives from her body (*soma*) and takes back in again, as tomb (*sema*). As seeds are planted, she is fertilized. She burgeons, gives fruit, and takes the seed in again during a stage of death and dormancy. A beautiful poetic fragment of this ritual cycle is expressed in the Sumerian Hymns to Inanna (Wolkstein and Kramer, 1983):

> Inanna spoke:
> My vulva, the horn, The
> Boat of Heaven,
> Is full of eagerness like the young moon.
> My untilled land lies fallow.
>
> As for me, Inanna,
> Who will plow my vulva? Who
> will plow my high field?
> Who will plow my wet ground?
>
> Dumuzi sang:
> O lady, your breast is your field.
> Inanna, your breast is your field.
> Your broad field pours out plants.
> Your broad field pours out grain.
> Water flows from on high for your servant.

Bread flows from on high for your servant.
Pour it out for me, Inanna.
I will drink all you offer.
(The Courtship of Inanna, pp. 27, 29)

The world is endlessly cyclical, and immortality is conceived in the repetition of the seasons and the tribe. Traditional cultures see themselves as fully intertwined with seasonal cycles. In ancient Greek, even the word for "bone marrow" was the same as the word for "wheat," and the words for young men and women were etymologically close to the word for "the shoots of young plants" (Kerenyi, 1967, p. 209). Blood was spattered on the field that the crops might grow. Tribal culture, whenever it made a sacrifice, considered it as a sacrament, feeling itself one with what was sacrificed and engaging in ritual mourning at its loss and death, but always knowing that life would return. Thus, it was easy to connect the life cycles of plants and animals with the life cycles of the tribe.

The ritual dances in which the tribe celebrated, invoked, and imitated cycles of the death and rebirth of the crops, according to Harrison, also celebrated the taking of the male child from its mother and initiating it into the tribal structure, where he eventually would become an elder and perform the same rites until he could no longer dance, at which point he would leave the tribe to die. This initiation was ritualized as a death-and-rebirth sequence. It was often accompanied with graphic re-enactments of birth, for example, by having a young man ceremonially killed and then jump through a goat skin smeared with blood to the noise of bull roarers:

> This pantomime, this pretended killing of the child, this painting him with clay and bringing him back to life again as a young man, is everywhere enacted. Till the boy has died and come to life again, till he has utterly 'put away childish things' he cannot be a full member of the tribe. ... Henceforth he belongs to something bigger, more potent, more lasting than his own individual existence: he is part of the stream

> of the totemic life, one with the generations before and yet to come.
>
> (Harrison 1962b, p. 19)

The tribal dancers, already initiated young men, wore white gypsum and were called *daimones* because they brought the spirits of the ancestors into the group. They became, in fact, the tribal ancestors as soon as they donned the gypsum. The initiates were sometimes compelled through the intensity of these rituals to forget entirely their childhood life, to forget their own name and acquire a new one, to forget how to speak and even sometimes not to recognize their mothers.

Part of the extraordinary sanctions of these rituals occurred because women as birth givers in ancient societies were feared as well as oppressed:

> She is charged with powers of child-bearing denied to man, powers only half understood, forces of attractions, but also of danger and repulsion, forces that all over the world seem to fill him with dim terror.
>
> (Harrison, 1962b, p. 36)

Harrison suggests that this experience can be imagined on both a microcosmic and macrocosmic level. The jolt of leaving the mother's world of nourishment to join the tribe as a warrior can be compared on a psychological level to the difficulty of leaving the mother's womb or the mother's breast to move out into the world, and then to become self-sufficient in whatever society is presented to one. The ritual can also express metaphorically the increasing gap between a world that worshipped the mother as a goddess of birth and death, and one that found such worship no longer necessary in the complexities of a civic world where the father appeared more essential. From mother-child unit to child alone, from mother earth to father sky, from matriliny and the tribe to patriliny and the patriarchal city-state, Harrison claims some such progression occurred.

The similes used in Homer's *Iliad* express a world of peace left behind that is decidedly pastoral and agricultural. There are as well numerous references suggestive of matriliny and matricentric culture in both the *Odyssey* and the *Iliad* (cf. Sculley, 1962; Butterworth, 1970). The story of Meleager in the *Iliad* hints as well of early ritual connected with the mother as earth. Hypothetical as such evidence, it is suggestive of what might lie in the heroic past.

Harrison's description of how traditional peoples related to the sacred is also evocative in considering the interaction of the Homeric hero with his gods. Harrison suggests that the creation of gods came about as human beings extended their own energies into the cosmos. When it was seen that tools could extend a person's power and effectiveness in the world, the tool took on a power of its own, as an extension of the personality of the person wielding it.

> What do we mean by the word sacred? ... In bygone days the answer would have been prompt and simple, the thunderbolt is sacred because it belonged to a god. The god is presupposed and from him comes the sanctity. We now know, from a study of the customs and representations of primitive peoples that, broadly speaking, the reverse is true, a thing is regarded as sacred, and out of that sanctity, given certain conditions, emerges a *daimon* and ultimately a god.

As Harrison tells us:

> *Le sacré, c'est le père du dieu.*
> "The sacred is the father of god."
>
> (1962b, p. 63)

When the tool's effectiveness was seen, it was worshipped. Harrison shows many early pictures of double axes, or so-called thunderstones, lying on altars. Later seal stones and reliefs show the same double axes, now wielded by the thunder god, Zeus. The same thing happened with powerful totem animals, such as the bull and the snake, out of which grew gods with bull's heads, and heroes with snake's tails.

Engaging in the celebration of their own sacred energy, their *mana*, in the dance, and worshipping tools and animals as extensions of themselves were different aspects of the same experience. Harrison notes that the individual in a tribe has

> a thin and meagre personality. If he dances alone, he will not dance long; but if his whole tribe dances together he will dance the live-long night and his emotion will mount to passion to ecstasy ... Emotion socialized, felt collectively, is emotion intensified and rendered permanent.
>
> (1962b, p. 43)

The undifferentiated collective emotion of the group as it gathered in dance to celebrate the rituals of the seasons gradually became concentrated in the *megistos daimon*, or chief dancer, as he marked himself off in the talent and energy from the rest of the group. Originally the tribe danced to celebrate and reflect (although perhaps not to effect). But the emergence of the seeds in spring, and the emergence of the *megistos daimon* in the dance brought about the attribution of a more and more differentiated personality of mana that came to be depicted as heroes and gods.

Gradually, as societies and personalities differentiated, gods became rather distant personalities to be worshipped, no longer a part of the energy of the dance, and men took part in a more political arena, leaving the natural gods, Dionysus, and mother earth, either on the outskirts or at the hearth of the cities, while they carried on the primary business of the world without them. The form of social structure based on the family and probably matrilineal, transformed to patrilineal, patriarchal rule. It is this that leads to their demise: "The Olympians are the last product of rationalism – cut off from the very source of their life and being, the emotion of the *thiasos* (band of worshippers). They desiccate and die" (Harrison, 1962b, p. 48).

Harrison's sense is that we move from a collectively held mana-filled world in which the desire of the worshipper gives birth to the gods to a collective *mana* that is increasingly differentiated.

As she says, "this vague force in man and in almost everything is constantly trembling on the verge of personality" (Harrison, 1962b, p. 67). Eventually gods are created and become personified as art forms. In so doing, they become cool and unconnected as they are personified and given human bodies. They no longer have *mana*, the vital substance ("libido" in a modern terminology) that holds us emotionally charged and webbed with the world. Harrison connects this depletion with the loss of connection to tribe and mother/matriliny/family.

If we follow Harrison, we can see mother earth writ large on a cosmos from whom we apparently must separate to become initiated into a tribe with its own separate responsibilities and consequently to be filled with rage that we cannot continue to live in Her sacred space. Were we to see the heroic world through a Harrisonian lens, we might say that the Olympian gods in Homer are certainly not yet abstract concepts; they are filled with *mana*. But neither does Homeric society seem to be the tightly knit world of Harrison's original tribal structure. This society is in the space of transition. That transition is fraught with ambivalence and the rage that accompanies loss.

In her framing of the evolution of cultures in this particular developmental sequence, Harrison echoes other 19th-century scholars such as Briffault in *The Mothers* (1977) and Bachofen in *Myth, Religion and Mother Right* (1967). She also inspires the work of psychologists who will speak of child development as a progression to a state of independence and autonomy. When she speaks of tools as extensions of personality and of the emanation of mana from the collective group, her thoughts are hauntingly suggestive of the way in which Winnicott will later define the transitional object. Like Winnicott's "blanket," the tool acquires the projected energy from the male tribal member to give it the magical quality of being an extension of himself, while at the same time connecting him powerfully to his functional world. This transitional quality makes him feel that he lives in a force field of *mana*, or of the sacred energy, which will eventually develop for him into the creation of gods. Harrison says that this event of the creation of gods is coincidental with the event of personality.

Personality arises as community organization gives birth to human beings noted for their superior abilities, and hence different from the group. Around this human being is developed a heroic narrative, which begins the development toward a sense of the individual. Consciousness of the linearity of time is developed as well, along with legendary histories that are specific, if not to individuals, then at least to individuals as the heroes of the specific families and communities. The gods then come to exist in time as reflections of the new sense of difference and individuality projected on to the cosmos from sources beyond ourselves, of which consciousness is at first unaware. Through visualizing, as in a mirror, the gods we create, we image ourselves as selves with increasing consciousness and integrity. Harrison here seems to be anticipating psychologists who emphasize the importance of mirroring on the part of the mother if one is to develop personality. Yet as the gods became affectively distanced, like parents left behind, Harrison, like Nietzsche, mourns their death. She regrets the autonomous, unemotional Cartesian self of her Enlightenment England and seeks to return to a mana-filled world that celebrated the nature god, Dionysus, where eponymous heroes still had snakes' tails. This mana-filled world, however, was not the same thing for her as oceanic bliss or fusion with the mother. It was a *transitional space* where the tribe danced and celebrated the seasons, perhaps just preceding the age of war in which the Homeric heroes lived together with their Olympians. Perhaps the very moment of attaining the conscious awareness that would eventually dispense with the Olympians came in the hero's *aristeia*, when he was fighting at his very best on the battlefield, like Harrison's *megistos kouros* leading the ritual dance. In both worlds, flashes of self-consciousness broke through a life lived immersed in magical connection with the cosmos.

When we consider the development of a culture extending from a matricentric tribal environment through a transitional period and then into a place of independence and autonomy where the fully interiorized self can flourish, we tend to think along linear, evolutionary lines. We also tend to think linearly about the world of the mother-infant dyadic relation that unfolds through a transitional period into the perception of self in a separate environment. But in both of these developmental sequences, time is never really linear any more than space is literal space. Time folds back on itself in such a way that any of these stages can be layered or interspersed with one another. Flashes of self-perception occur in the opaqueness of a merged environment, and transitions can be experienced almost simultaneously as the peace and serenity of play and as a space of sudden and violent ambivalence and the fear of loss.

Sociological evidence joins Harrisonian hypotheses in agreeing that the period of the Trojan War shows many strains involved in the movement from a family-oriented to a political world (Seaford, 1995). One of the greatest of these is the danger involved in patriliny. As soon as the child begins to take the father's name, and as soon as it is important to the father to carry on his ancestral line, given that he is no longer part of the intimate tribal unit, the father must be assured that his son is his own. The only way this can occur is if he keeps his wife/woman close to him. If she is stolen, his line is bastardized, and his very immortality is in danger. Both in hunter/gatherer and in agricultural societies immortality is not important, because the world is lived in repetitive sacred cycles. But as soon as personality differentiation begins to develop, it becomes clear that one's immortality can only be carried on by one's own progeny and one's own glory. Loss of women, therefore, as shown in the Trojan War, is well worth fighting about, not just because guest friendship has been betrayed, not because women are priceless booty, but because the hero's very sense of identity and immortality depends on them.

In a mortal, heroic universe, it is essential that the gods are deathless and ageless rather than cyclical like the seasons over which Dionysus, the wild, nature god presides (and who is mentioned only once in the *Iliad*). The more defined and separate the personality becomes, as it copes with a cosmos that is relative and not fixed, and the more it feels disjointed from community and family, the more stress will be placed on maintaining a separate individuality, and the more difficulty there will be with the notion of maintaining permeability. Connective tissues between gods, nature, and community encourage permeability and have it as an unspoken regulatory system. It appears that the very rules of reciprocity and revenge are the boundaries that make permeability possible. Within that context there can be flow. When relationships become more flexible and less bounded by the unwritten and sacred customs of family and tribe, then there is also more tendency to breakdown and conflict, and one must keep oneself more protectively bounded.

7.2 Homeric Heroes and Matricentrism

However we stand in relation to the issue of whether or not Jung's and Neumann's belief that the childhood of a race and the childhood of an infant human being are in any way parallel, or that the psychological-mythological stages experienced in their respective development are similar, their ideas are evocative in the light of other evidence that the permeability of the heroic psyche is dependent upon the notion of a tightly inter-webbed, matricentric community that is based on tribal and familial values rather than civic governance. The psyche it spawns is not individuated, coherent, or bounded as it is in our world. Many of the Homeric heroes are quixotic and undependable in temperament, raging at one moment and weeping at the next. Their moods and states of being are multiple and usually are not influenced by any sense of personal judgment. From a modern perspective, their communications with gods, lapses of perception, and inability to conduct themselves in an orderly fashion appear to fall under the description of hallucinatory and dissociative behaviors. Indeed, they are not unlike our so-called "borderline" personalities, who live perilously on the edges of fantasy and reality and can experience no stability of mood because they have little internalized sense of self.

But Homeric heroes, unlike borderline personalities trying to survive in our western sociopolitical structures, live and function well in their own familial and tribal societies and find resilience in immortal connection. Achilles, the one hero who cannot be reasoned with at all and who insists on living outside the dominant tribal code and under the auspices of his divine mother, appears mad. Yet, interestingly, he alone discovers the meaning of compassion and a more individual justice through mourning.

When Achilles and Priam come together in Priam's asking for Hector's body, rules of the suppliant and of guest friendship must be obeyed. Yet Achilles has rarely followed these rules. He is dangerous in his emotional outbursts; he fights with an intensity and a cruelty that far exceed that of either god or beast. In the exchange with Priam, he holds to the rules by what seems to be a thread:

> Don't stir my raging heart still more.
> Or under my own roof I may not spare your life, old man – suppliant that you are – may break the laws of Zeus!
> (Homer, 1990, R. Fagles, trans., *Il.* 24, 667–670)

It is Achilles' very emotional movement beyond the communal structures he knows, however, that leads him to see that Priam, a man the age of his own father, is mourning the death of his beloved son, as he himself is mourning the death of a beloved. And it is their grieving together that brings empathy into the world, an empathy that deepens and begins to interiorize the psyche. Here, there is a genuine metaphorical exchange, in which Achilles understands that even though he is face to face with the father of the very man whose son killed his beloved Patroclus, both of them share the same grief. It is this kind of hero who can see into the specific character of a given human being and arrange the chariot race in the funeral games according to the justice that is personally appropriate for each driver. Personality here moves beyond tribe into the judging of the qualities of each hero individually, and then into building an order of justice accordingly. Unfortunately, however, the ending harmony of the *Iliad* is not to be recapitulated in most of the journeys home, where familial disobedience and hatred reign.

The only two Greek heroes who do manage to achieve some sense of "home," metaphorically as well as literally, are Achilles and Odysseus. Curiously, these are the two heroes most connected and responsive to women, whether as mothers, wives, or lovers. Achilles, although he will be shot in his heel with a poisoned arrow by Paris and not make it home, has already heard through a long and touching dialogue with his divine mother Thetis, as he weeps by the seashores of Troy, that he is fated to a live a short but glorious life (Homer, 1990, *Il.* I. 413–500). His rage is over the stealing of his woman, Briseis, who always appears to have more value to him than property or mere possessions. Through his mourning over Patroclus and the reparation achieved with Priam, he has evoked a sense of justice in himself and in his small world of the funeral games.

Odysseus ultimately returns home to Penelope, but only after ten years of wandering, at the end of which Calypso also finds him weeping by the shore and sends him to the underworld. Here he sees his mother and desperately tries to hold her in his arms, only to find that she is without substance and cannot be held, but only fades into the distance:

> And I, my mind in turmoil, how I longed
> to embrace my mother's spirit, dead as she was!
> Three times I rushed toward her, desperate to hold her,
> like a shadow, dissolving like a dream, and each time the
> grief cut to the heart, sharper, yes, and I,
> I cried out to her, words winging into the darkness:
> "Mother, why not wait for me?"
>
> (Homer, 1996, R. Fagles, trans. [*Od.* Xl., 233–240])

Odysseus' landing on the magical island of Phaeacia almost makes him a wedding partner for Nausicaa until he, weeping, retells his own story and expresses his longing to return home. There is even a suggestion that Odysseus is doubly born from a woman, in that Nausicaa finds him naked and wrapped in dirt and leaves and brings him to "birth" on shores of the island. This stands in stark contrast to being born a second time through the process of initiation into the male tribal-civic structure of which Harrison speaks.

Both Achilles and Odysseus are more connected to their mother than other Greek heroes, and simultaneously find union and resolution through actions that suggest a more defined, integral self. It is possible that heroes who remain close to their mothers, who do not rip themselves away or find themselves ripped ultimately away, are better able to remain in what we have defined as expanded transitional space. Once again, the ability to grieve allows the insight that can maintain positive connections to living in a webbed world, without the heroic separation that Neumann says must involve "killing the monster."

Erich Neumann, Melanie Klein, and Jane Harrison, although they differ considerably in their descriptions of how transitional space is negotiated, appear to be in agreement that the transition out of either the mother or the matricentric culture is achieved only with tremendous ambivalence and violence. Neumann speaks of the dragon slayer, Klein of the instinctual aggressive drive and, metaphorically, of biting the good breast, and Harrison of the actual enacted violence in initiation ceremonies of second birth. If we set the *Iliad* in such a contest of transition from a matricentric to a patriarchal society, parallel to the development of the infant as described in the language of these three authors, the rage and aggression of its heroes become more understandable.

Kohut (1977, 1984) and Bollas (1987) are far less concerned with the necessity of separation from the mother into a place of radical autonomy where the ego must act as a lone and entirely self-sustaining hero. They do not see transitional space simply as a space to move through, but rather as a sustainable, endlessly creative space of intrinsic worth and value. They see a natural assertiveness in the infant that with good-enough, careful nourishment from the mother can then develop the maternal idiom and selfobject connections, blossoming into increasingly wider creative webs throughout life. They would undoubtedly see the transition to a place of autonomy and independence where the gods are merely "objets d'art" as involving a great loss for the individual (hero).

Achilles and Odysseus do not give up their mothers but stay close to the connected and emotional "feminine" throughout their lives. Achilles weeps by the shore and takes advice from his semi-divine mother Leto, which renders him able through his grief over his beloved Patroclus to show empathy for Priam. Odysseus mourns his mother in the underworld and, through his love for his wife, Penelope, is able to return home. Neither appear to need such radical separation as leaving their mothers fully behind in order to become individuals.

Perhaps living in and valuing a world of expanded transitional space, as I have defined it in relation to the Homeric hero, has something to do with the extent to which the hero can stay in touch and connection with the mother while still expanding his webs of experience. Perhaps it also has to do with the extent to which we are willing to recognize the potential of a community to hold some self for us, a community engaging nature and the sacred to which we can return after we have developed sufficient self-consciousness to symbolize, interpret, and feel at home with ourselves.

7.3 Conclusion

Harrison, Neumann, Klein, and Winnicott, even in their efforts to describe transitional space, bind themselves in languages of projection and introjection, inside and outside, thereby reinforcing the very boundaries they seek to displace. All are deeply engaged with the world of mother and the development into either a personal or a cultural adulthood.

Harrison herself, influenced by both Jung and Freud, makes such statements as "divinity at its very source is human" (1962b, p. 47), and "the awful, the uncanny, the unknown is within man rather than without" (p. 65), thereby showing that she too begins within the human being and moves outward, assuming that the forces in the cosmos are all the result of our projections. This is not what the heroic worldview believed, or the way heroes lived. The concept of projection is the linguistic product of a world that is no longer in a state of webbed consciousness, but perhaps wishes it were.

The challenge for psychotherapeutic healers concerned with contemporary formulations of an intersubjective, multiple self, or with creating or acknowledging an atmosphere in the therapy room that is intersubjective, is to see how far and in what ways we are willing to acknowledge psychic permeability as a criterion for health before we believe it to become destructive in nature. How strong a hold must we have on the subject-object relationship before we allow ourselves to flow with others or to let down our self-structures to allow whatever gods and demons choose to knock, to enter? The Homeric world encourages us to believe that the archaic psyche may still have imaginal and vibrant vitality, despite its inherent madness and potential for disintegration. It may still call us to a place where what we may feel as aggressive and dissociative behavior can be tolerated, indeed welcomed, if held in the cradle of a therapeutic, maternal surround. Homer's *Iliad* itself, of course, is an aesthetic creation that has the capacity, as art, to heal the soul.

References

Bachofen, J.J. (1967). *Myth, Religion, & Mother Right: Selected Writings of J.J. Bachofen* (R. Mannheim, trans.) Princeton, NJ: Princeton University Press.

Bollas, C. (1987). *The Shadow of the Object: Psychoanalysis of the Unthought Known.* New York: Columbia University Press.

Briffault, R. (1977). *The Mothers.* New York: Atheneum.

Butterworth, E.A.S. (1970). *The Tree at the Navel of the Earth.* Berlin, Germany: De Gruyter.

Cornford, F. (1912). *From Religion to Philosophy.* London: Arnold.

Eigen, M. (1996). *Psychic Deadness.* Northvale, NJ: Jason Aronson.

Frazer, J.G. (1911–15). *The Golden Bough: A Study in Magic and Religion* (Vols. 1–12). London: McMillan & Co.

Harrison, J.E. (1962a). *Epilegomena to the Study of Greek Religion and Themis: A Study of the Social Origins of Greek Religion.* New York: University Books.

Harrison, J.E. (1962b). *Themis: A Study of the Social Origins of Greek Religion.* Cleveland: Meridian Press.

Homer (1990). *The Iliad* (Robert Fagles, trans.). New York: Viking Penguin.

Homer (1996). *The Odyssey* (Robert Fagles, trans.). New York: Penguin Putnam.

Jaynes, J. (1976). *The Origins of Consciousness in the Breakdown of the Bicameral Mind.* Boston, MA: Houghton Mifflin Company.

Kohut, H. (1977). *The Restoration of the Self.* New York: International Universities Press.

Kohut, H. (1984). *How Does Analysis Cure?* (A. Goldberg and P. Stepansky, eds.). Chicago: Chicago University Press.

Murray, G. (1955). *Five Stages of Greek Religion.* Garden City, NY: Doubleday.

Neumann, E. (1973). *The Origins and History of Consciousness* (3rd ed.). Princeton: Princeton University Press.

Plato (1961). *The Republic*. In Hamilton and Cairns (eds.), *The Collected Dialogues of Plato.* New York: Pantheon Books.

Sculley, V.T. (1962). *The Earth, the Temple, and the Gods*. New Haven, CT: Yale University Press.

Seaford, R. (1995). *Reciprocity and Ritual: Homer and Tragedy in the Developing City-State.* New York: Oxford University Press.

Snell, B. (1960). *The Discovery of the Mind* (T.G. Rosenmeyer, trans.). Oxford: Oxford University Press. (Original work published 1953.)

Thucydides (1951). *The Peloponnesian War* (J.H. Finley, Jr., ed.). Modem Library: New York.

Wolkstein, D. and Kramer, S.N. (1983). *Inanna: Queen of Heaven and Earth.* New York: Harper & Row.

Chapter 8

The Birth of the Subject in Aeschylus

8.1 From Epic to Drama

Aeschylus' *Oresteia* is a profoundly transformative work for ancient Greek culture in that it embodies the shift from a ritual and communal to a legal and civic worldview, centering in the creation of the democratic city-state of Athens in the mid-5th century BCE. Aeschylus is the earliest of the tragedians whose work remains to us in any integrity. Through his *Oresteia*, in particular, we can observe how this shift from a ritual, nonpersonal view of the cosmos gave way to the sense of a nascent subject who was to become the citizen of a city-state, separate from mother, family, and tribal community. Such a move marks a turning point in ancient Greek culture. The *Oresteia* was first produced in 458 BCE just as the city-state of Athens was becoming a full democracy, Pericles reigned, and the Acropolis was built.

The breakdown of huge, communal, archetypal forces into discrete political and legal processes is epitomized in Aeschylus' language, which moves in its style from a monumental architecture of compounded words with bare traces of grammar, viscous and metaphorically dense in the *Agamemnon*; to the magical language of the dirge that calls up Agamemnon's ghost to assist the children Orestes and Electra in plotting the death of their mother, in the *Libation Bearers*, to the simple, legalistic, rhetorical, and persuasive language of the *Eumenides*, which finally acquits Orestes. The change in language reveals a transformation of the Greek psyche, the foundational psyche for the western world.

This encapsulated transformation of language is highly evocative of the development of the infant from a fused,

DOI: 10.4324/9781003340751-10

pre-metaphorical unity within its mother world, through transitional space, to a moment in which it can become aware of itself as a symbolizing creature. In the transformation from a matricentric to patriarchal world, we can recognize much of what Freud, Klein, and other psychoanalysts centuries later are going to interpret in psychic development as a shift from primary identification to secondary process formulations.

Before entering into a discussion of how this works in the *Oresteia* in detail, it will be helpful to look at the meaning and function of ancient Greek Tragedy in its historical and ritual context. The tragic heroes of Greek drama are taken from Homer's *Iliad* and *Odyssey*, as well as from other heroic sagas dating from about 300 years prior to the so-called Golden Age of Athens. The heroes themselves celebrated in the epics had existed in tribal memory for as long as 400 years prior to their composition. The classical Greeks lived and breathed with these heroes, celebrating their legendary ancestry. However, the shift from the tribal world to the world of complex politics in the Athenian *polis* was tremendous, and drama cast epic heroes on the stage for the populace to see, to all appearances still Homeric, yet caught in and suffering the throes of the new and unrecognizable world in which their social structure, beliefs, and values were no longer effective. The permeable psyches of the epic heroes, which once could live within their flexible boundaries, had fallen under siege.

8.2 Ritual Origins of Greek Tragedy

The word "drama" emerges from the word *dromenon*, or "ritual." Ritual, to recapitulate Harrison's view, is a sacramental act, with the intent of gathering *mana* (sacred energy). Often a dance, the ritual celebrates the cycling of the seasons through time (see Chapter 7 for a full discussion). The *dromenon* was an act "predone" in anticipation of the new year, "done" in immediate identification with the seasonal cycle, and "redone" to mimic the ritual that had been done from time immemorial.

This pre-doing, doing, and redoing of the cosmos in ritual is an act of *mimesis*. It mirrors the movements of the cosmos, as the cosmos mirrors that of human beings. In the mirroring itself, the world comes into being. At first, tools and animals are worshipped as extensions of personality that make the tribe one with the sacred mana of the world. The ritual is primary in calling forth the pity and suffering through the sacrificing of the animal felt to be a part of the tribe's identity. The tribal person ingests that animal to share in its sacredness, thus becoming one with it, the community, and the seasonal cycles. Through identification with the sacrifice in its dying and rebirthing arises the experience of purification or catharsis. Without this act, life cannot proceed. As peoples gradually come to realize that mana can be manipulated and begin to sense their difference and their power as human beings as distinct from plants and animals, first heroes and then the Olympian gods are born, mirroring newfound capacities and awareness of human functions. Nevertheless, the tribe is still aware of itself as part of the world's natural processes. There is as yet no clear perception of self, self-determination, or the vaguest of senses that one can choose one's destiny apart from the tribe. The recognition in the enactment of the ritual of present celebration, gratitude for the past, and anticipation of the future engages an awareness of time in which as one awaits and celebrates a sacred that is present in the moment, one is simultaneously aware of moments past and anticipated. In the liminality of such moments, both art and religion are born: "If we are utterly, instantly satisfied, if we were a mass of well-contrived instincts, we should have no representations, no memory, no *mimesis*, no *dromena*, no drama. Art and religion alike spring from unsatisfied desire" (Harrison, 1962a, p. 44). This "unsatisfied desire" formulates itself as a desire for meaning.

Greek Tragedy is an art form that emerged from this ritual way of thinking and believing. Dionysus himself was its chief priest. Performances took place in the spring, a time when the seas became calm, when foreigners, islanders, and those who lived on the mainland outside of Athens could gather in the city. The Great Dionysia, as it was called, was open to all (except possibly Athenian women) and was both profoundly religious and political in nature. The Athenian audience participated in it with great emotion and intensity. Aristotle, in his definitive work on tragedy, *The Poetics*, written in the 4th century BCE, tells us that the best tragedies were able to produce pity and fear so deep as to affect the emotional catharsis and transformation that one would expect from rituals in which the people were not an audience, but active participants. Catharsis occurred through identification of the audience with the protagonist or tragic figure, and with his or her activities and sufferings. By suffering with the tragic hero, the audience could then experience their own catharsis, which enabled them to live again and to be reborn into the daily community.

It might seem that identification with a single character is suddenly astoundingly different from feeling a part of the tribal whole. True, the tragic hero was set apart from the chorus and did not appear to emanate from it. But, like the *megistos daimon* of the ritual, who was the most vital or mana-filled of the *titanes* (members of the tribe masked in white clay as their ancestors), the tragic hero gathered sacred energy. Like the *megistos daimon*, he was masked, and at the time of Aeschylus, the masks were generically formalized to represent gender and the ages of life but not much more. Masks were, in the Jungian sense, "personae." It was the "persona" that first began to allow for the containment of a personality out from the collective unconscious (Campbell, 1971, p. 97). Finally, it was not the tragic hero who determined the action. Plot determined character, not vice versa:

> The plot, then, is the principle and, as it were, the soul of tragedy: character comes second. In fact, there is a parallel even in painting: if some artist were to lay on the finest colors without order he would not delight the viewer as well as the artist who sketches the likeness of an object in black and white. Tragedy, after all, is an imitation of an action; and it is an imitation of agents for the sake of that action most of all (Aristotle, 1983, *Poetics* 1449a39–1450b4).

For Aristotle, then, character in the classical drama he was writing about is a kind of quality that influences action, but is not crucial to drama, because it does not inherently have order, nor can it make order. Rather, character is like tint or color added to painting. If character is that which imbues action, then it is action rather than the agent that creates the soul of tragedy. If this is so, then the order of the plot gives meaning to human beings, and characters are merely parts of the whole. In other words, agents themselves are not necessarily consistent or continuous beyond the context in which they occur, nor do they order the context. Character needs to be contextualized in order to have coherence and meaning. That is, character finds definition through process. It is not a "state" of being, the way we might define "self" as a state, as it if were something we could look at or define as a thing in itself. Indeed, as Aristotle says,

> Tragedy is an imitation not of men, but of action and a way of life … Hence performers act not in order to imitate character; they take on character for the sake of (imitating) actions … Besides, without action tragedy would not exist, but it would exist without character.
>
> (Aristotle, 1983, [*Arist.* 1450a, 16–25])

By action, Aristotle means the structured movement of the rise and fall of a tragic figure who is enough like us that we can identify with him or her, causing the pity and fear that bring about catharsis. In other words, Aristotle is defining a *dromenon* in which the tragic figure has now replaced the animal sacrifice. The catharsis which we share with this figure in his or her doom brings us to the awareness of our own doom. Through the emptying out of these feelings of pity and fear, the audience can be purified and reborn. It is not individual characters that are important – they are mere flavors and tints – but the action into which fate has thrust them.

Yet, tragic drama is a ritual structure in which the audience participates by viewing rather than dancing. In other words, the act of perception has replaced the act of participation, so the audience is experiencing from a perspective that is at one remove. It is this extraordinary change that first allows the possibility for the emergence of character and for the interiorizing of great cosmic forces. The very setting of the Athenian amphitheater, where one looks down from a great height onto tiny figures set against the actual landscape of the mountains and sea of Greece, where the plays are enacted. Beginning in the early morning and ending as the sun sets at once brings unity with landscape and the circling of time, as well as the beginning of a focus down and into psyche:

Tragedy is the concentrated, intense genre that its community prized, for which they shut up shop, came to their uncomfortable theater, and sat still for days on end. Its ways of looking at human beings and human relations with the outside world must have had some bearing on that community's inner life (Padel, 1992, p. 6).

In sum, ancient Greek drama embodied at its most fundamental and existential level the thoughts, beliefs, and concerns of its people. Its audience, although not dancing the ritual, were nevertheless active participants living an internal ritual in participation with others. As the *dromenon* mirrored the seasons, so did drama mirror the psyche. This still permeable psyche, set ritually within a performance context, may well presage the ritual moment of the interactive therapeutic setting.

8.3 Aeschylus' *Oresteia*

The *Oresteia* is a series of three plays, all of which were performed on a single day, from sunrise to sundown. It depicts the return of the great Argive King Agamemnon to his home after ten years, upon winning the Trojan war. On his return, he is killed by his wife, Clytemnestra. Because of a blood law that commands any relative to avenge the murder of kin, Orestes, Agamemnon's and Clytemnestra's son, is commanded by Apollo to kill his mother in recompense for his father's death. However, Orestes is unfortunately related to both his parents, therefore killing his mother for killing his father leaves him in the predicament of having killed a blood relation himself. The Furies, ancient goddesses and guarantors of the blood law, demand that Orestes be killed in turn, but Apollo saves Orestes with Athena's help by presenting his case in a legal trial at the Areopagus, the city law court.

At the trial, evidence is presented based on the precedent of the motherless Athena, who sprang fully armed from her father Zeus' head, that Orestes does not in fact carry the blood of his mother, because mothers are simply baskets who hold their young but do not contribute biologically to them. Thus, Orestes is acquitted by a single vote, a tie breaker by Athena, and the Furies after much persuasion agree to inhabit the underground beneath the Areopagus, to remain revered, but only in charge of birth, giving up their claim to the familial blood law of vengeance and revenge (a law we have seen more recently on screen in the Sicilian mafia world of the Godfather films).

As an historical text, the *Oresteia* documents the yielding of family law to state law, and the move from a matricentric to a patriarchal system. It also shows the move from the symbolic and magical language of curses, omens, and oracles to the rhetorically persuasive language of the law court, where not absolute commands of divine law but relative judgments hold sway. Protagoras is shortly to pronounce in the Athenian *agora* that man is the measure of all things, establishing with this statement that there are no fundamental, unshakeable truths, not even of biology. One man may be acquitted of his mother's murder; another may not. All has become relative, and the unchangeable orders of the ancient female gods as well as familial rights now seem to be written, like the words of women, as Sophocles says, on water.

Aeschylus is not unaware that the ripping apart of the web of a former belief system causes great psychic tragedy. Not only is there parental death, but, despite Orestes' acquittal, it is clear that he will be plagued with insanity. The breaking of familial law and the transformation of the Furies are fraught with ambivalence. Aeschylus, despite the father-focus in the medical literature of the time, was well aware of the mother world and the mother's contribution. The basis for the legal decision in the final play is in fact redolent with irony in that Aeschylus himself was presumably an initiate in the Eleusinian mysteries, which worshipped the seasonal, cyclic rituals overseen by Demeter and her daughter Persephone.

Aeschylus is difficult to read, whether in Greek or in English. His characters look like empty, two-dimensional figures on a cosmic screen in which the long lyrics of the choruses hold sway. Contemporary student audiences tend to become bored and frustrated when reading Aeschylus, whereas they do not when reading Euripides, the so-called first psychological tragedian. A closer look at our own cultural lens suggests that students may be bored with empty figures and complex lyrics heavy with symbolism but unconnected with inner selves. This is a tip-off to the fact that what we as modern audiences sense in his drama is a cultural moment in which the psyche appears to be two-dimensional in characterization because it is in fact not yet understood as a coherent self with internal functions. Character is still permeable, more a process than a state, highly influenced by outside forces (as were the epic heroes), and in fact defined through its connections with those outside forces. The gods, signs, and oracles through which these characters live might well be understood from our frame of reference as transitional phenomena which have not yet been internalized to form the coherent, bounded structure called self, which we have assumed to be a given.

Although Clytemnestra, in the first play of the trilogy, "Agamemnon," appears to choose to kill her husband, she at no point appears either engaged in the process of choosing or conflicted in her choice. Quite otherwise, she claims authority to do this act from ritual and divine sources, and as a proper sacrifice to the gods of the underworld. Many believe that Clytemnestra's claim that she killed Agamemnon for sacrificing their daughter Iphigenia to bring up the winds to sail to Troy is an excuse, and that in fact she acts out of a personal vendetta. But even if Clytemnestra may seem to act partly on her own behalf, she still does so as leader of the ancient goddesses, the Furies, and so as a primal ritual force empowered by a chthonic community. In other words, the power and agency with which Clytemnestra acts is not just personally considered and chosen but takes place according to a ritual law of retribution for crime committed against blood kin. Agamemnon has killed Iphigeneia, their daughter.

Agamemnon is at best cowardly in the face of his wife's greetings and demands. His choice to pollute the tapestries of the royal palace by walking on them is guided by his wife's rhetorical insistence, and constitutes a strong analogy to the ritual of the Bouphonia in which an ox is made to choose willingly to eat barley cakes from an altar before its sacrifice, thereby selecting itself as victim. Agamemnon's murder, then, bears all the marks of an animal sacrifice to cleanse pollution. It is hard to sympathize with his death, especially given the chorus' hidden, mutinous feelings toward him for conducting a long war in which many Greek youths and husbands were killed. Cassandra, the only other major figure in the *Agamemnon*, is fascinating as a mad prophetess, and inspires pathos as the figure caught in the webs of others' lives, condemned as prophetess never to be believed by her audience, but there is little internal character there as we know it.

The only trace of a real human relationship occurs in the second play, the *Choephori,* or *Libation Bearers*, between Electra, Orestes' sister, and Orestes himself, when they recognize each other after a long absence through the token of hair they have each put on their father's tomb. Yet even in this play, Orestes, as a son caught in the bind of a father-mother murder with moral obligations to kill his own mother, seems but the victim of external forces. It is Apollo who commands him to kill his mother. It is the Furies who will make boils burst out all over Orestes' skin and pursue him throughout Greece, visiting fits of madness upon him because he has committed matricide.

In the "*Eumenides*," the last play of the trilogy, it will be Athena who saves Orestes, through casting a vote for his acquittal. We want to know Orestes' inner agony, but it appears there is no inner. Aside from a moment of hesitation in which he asks his friend Pylades whether or not he should kill his mother, there appears to be little guilt and little remorse in him with which we can identify. Euripides is to fill out all these figures in his plays, 30 or so years later, and turn tragedy into psychological drama as we know it. Interestingly, the ancient Greek audience considered his plays melodramatic, and never awarded him first prize, perhaps suggesting that they still held to the motion of drama as communal ritual.

Where the transitional play space of the epic hero was the battlefield on which gods, divine forces, nature and heroes all struggled together, the transitional space of drama of the *Agamemnon* describes a liminal world where human beings are specks and pawns, held in the grip of massive, inescapable forces. These tiny figures are no longer in direct communication with their gods. No tragic hero, like Achilles, was seized by the hair and admonished by Athena, nor could Helen arrogantly mock Aphrodite by telling her to go lie with Paris herself, if she loved him so much. Rather, the gods spoke through oracles, signs, and omens cast against a distant sky, which could be interpreted only by prophets and seers; gods spoke in the darkness of dreams, which frequently could be divined, except that in this world, fear grew so great in the chaos of the gods receding that sleep itself gave way to sleeplessness. As the night watchman says, waiting for the signal of Troy's defeat on his rooftop for ten full years:

> And when I keep my couch that sends me wandering by night, my couch wet with dew, this couch of mine that no dreams visit –/ for Fear of Sleep stands by it, so that I may not close my eyes fast in sleep –
>
> (Aeschylus, 1979, trans. H. Lloyd-Jones, [*Aesch. Ag.* 12–15])

Families and laws of reciprocity and guest friendship had been defiled by the exigencies of war, even after the Greeks had won the Trojan War. The god Ares had brought back jars of dust instead of living husbands. They did not balance in the scales of war or justice (cf. Aeschylus, 1979). In Agamemnon's home of Argos, resentment grew against the leader who had killed his own daughter to spark the winds to sail to Troy and had left Clytemnestra, her mother, to fuel her vengeance in the ten bitter years he had left his palace empty. His action had put state over family, depriving mothers of their birthright and rightful location at the center of the tribe, as the raiser and protector of children and the priestesses of sacred, seasonal cycles.

We have seen that in the epic world, heroes felt themselves to be permeable and multiple rather than contained and cohesive. The fluid that ran through their bodies created their organs; their psyches were not individual souls, but breath that moved in and out of them, and flew from them at death: each of their organs was inhabited by a different god, making them more closely connected in their various parts to multiple divine forces than to any sense of inner integrity. Objects and elements in the world around the heroes were also seen as extensions of themselves, and they themselves became part of their accoutrements. Language itself was not mere empty abstraction, but formed fluid substance, connecting heroes with nature, community, and divine. Words themselves sang heroes into everlasting glory – the poet's speech was truth, "the absence of forgetfulness," formed of honey, of dew. Theirs was a neither-nor space, lived in a webbed flow with the cosmos, where flashes of self-consciousness were experienced in the intense, exalted moments of a hero's *aristeia* (his most glorious moment) as he battled another to the death on a field where heroes, gods and natural forces thrashed and crashed together in a crucial, death-defying play that would ultimately birth the consciousness of otherness and interiority.

Aeschylean tragedy, in contrast, while expressing a similar view of the psyche's permeability, thunders with grand, elemental forces that pour through his language in the form of omens, signs, and oracles. They shiver and crack the *phrenes*, "lungs-mind" (cf. Onians, 1951) of the tragic heroes, rendering their sense of permeability with the cosmos terrifyingly out of control. Tragic heroes become vulnerable in their lack of cohesion and in their attempt to rely on overarching cosmic laws. The body pours its liquids out in tears, blood, and the yellow liquids of death. Life itself in the old men of the chorus in the *Agamemnon* is as fragile and brittle as falling leaves. We are more aware of the flow of processes of life, death, and time passing than of any solidity or stability. The balance has tipped. Fear and Age are elemental forces huge in comparison to human beings and inflict their sufferings upon them. The air is thick with forces, divinities, and symbols more substantial than humans themselves. The tragic actor wears a mask twice as large as his face and covering his head completely, bearing a single, agonized expression through which these forces flow.

It is as if the conflicts and emotional traumas that we believe interior to ourselves are cast all over the cosmos, extending as far as the canopy of stars, caught and spreading through the fires of the torchlight leaping from mountain to mountain carrying the news of Greek victory from Troy to Argos. These fires, of funeral pyres and of the burning city ignite murderous rage in Clytemnestra and hot madness in Cassandra. It is not Clytemnestra's rage or Cassandra's madness. It is fire itself that is incendiary and all consuming. Its individual manifestations in rage, sickness, evil, and madness are but the single flames of a giant holocaust. It is, as Heraclitus says, at once one and many. We cannot claim our emotions or actions as emanating from within us, nor can we tolerate their externality. They strike us from without. The gods and forces have impelled us. This sense of fragility is in itself a recognition that there is no longer a tribe to sustain, a ritual to keep order or to grant communal immortality. Tragic figures are alone and mortal in a shattered, postwar world.

This is a world in which the transformation of language effects and affects the interiorization and recognition of self. Omens and signs move from the space of the external heavens into rich and internalized symbolic metaphors. As signs remain omens while also taking on symbolic resonances, they appear to control the dramatic action, sweeping it along with tragic and unalterable consequences to the characters. The entire Aeschylean cosmos in the *Agamemnon* is enmeshed in imprisoning ambivalence.

The omen of the eagles and hare that the old men read in the sky at the beginning of the *Agamemnon* appears as the encompassing symbol in whose structure all action is identified and frozen, endlessly repeating itself. This omen is expressed in the oppositional language of the Delphic Oracle, which at once gives it validity and brings it to effective birth in the world.

Simultaneously, this oppositional language mirrors the eternal laws themselves, which although appropriate for a world of the ritual tribe that reveres seasonal cycles and does not fear mortality because it does not recognize itself as composed of mortal individuals, is devastating for a world that is bringing individuals into being and is all too aware of the mortality of such beings. In other words, while the omen brings what is felt into clarity through oppositional language, the oppositions simultaneously freeze the action, allowing the characters no possibility for a choice that goes beyond them.

The simultaneous clarifying of conflicts and situating of ambivalences strongly evoke a Kleinian world, where the infant, an enmeshed creature with disorganized needs, tries to organize his world into good and bad through projective-introjective splitting, in this way attaining what Klein calls the paranoid-schizoid position. Without this original, oppositional splitting into good and bad, there is no hope for the Kleinian infant to move through the paranoid-schizoid position into the depressive and then finally reparative stages. Instead of breaking through oppositional symbols into a more flexible, individuated paradoxical language that might give the participants in the drama some understanding of themselves as interpreting subjects who might then be free themselves from imprisoning splits, the possibility of the development of the subject is halted, and oppositions as well as cosmic, parental authorities are clung to all the more strongly.

We see this occurring in the second play in *Oresteia*, the "Choephori," where, obedient to Apollo's command to Orestes and Electra, the children of Agamemnon, call up his ghost in a magically binding dirge to help them to slaughter their mother. Klein interrupts this act of murder and Orestes' consequent remorse for it as the attainment of the depressive position by Orestes (Klein, 1940/1963). However, the legal, rhetorical language of the last play, the *Eumenides*, which is singularly non-symbolic and without oracular style except as manipulative technique on Athena's part, suggests that no depressive position is reached. That Orestes goes insane and continues to be pursued by the Furies even after his legal acquittal also suggests that agency and integrity have not been achieved. Rather, we see the creation of a fragile, non-resilient self in Orestes, who tries to attain autonomy without any connection to the mother world while simultaneously denying himself as a symbolizing subject. In sum, unlike Winnicott's conceptualization of transitional space as birthing the symbolizing being, or Klein's formulation of the paranoid-schizoid position yielding through guilt to the depressive and then reparative positions, the legal resolution in the *Eumenides* is formulated in such a way that the mother is entirely erased as giving any of her genetic material to the infant, and the need for the sacred is repressed and driven underground with the Furies. Athena, the only residue of the female – a virgin born fully armed from her father, Zeus' head – is in no way in charge of birth and generation, but is rather a military figurehead for the Athenian city-state.

8.3.1 Omens and Ambivalence: The First Chorus

The chorus of elders at the beginning shows that cosmic processes of time and being are far more dominant and overriding than human character, and that human beings are entirely subject to eternal laws. But they also show how the very interpretation of divine signs lends prophetic authority through their oracular phrasing. Such phrasing both brings the formlessness of the cosmos into distinction, allowing it to become clear within the context of the familiar order of talion law, and binds the actors to re-enact its patterns. Uttered language brings the hidden to light and the ineffective to effectiveness. We are held in a space where physical form and definition are emerging from the flowing processes of a permeable cosmos, yet at the same time fading back into them. Humanity is tenuous, scarcely able to retain its distinctness – a state analogous to the prelinguistic stage of early infant fusion with the mother in psychology, except that this mother reflects the maternal, ritual cosmos. This is how the old men describe themselves:

> For the fresh stuff of life that within the breast holds sway is like an old man's and the war god is not as his post; and great

> age with the leaf already withering on three feet walks, and with strength no greater than a child's like a dream seen by day wanders.
>
> (Aeschylus, 1979 [Aesch. *Ag*. 78–82]).

At each moment of description, it is not the old men who are the subjects. It is the "stuff of life" within that is the subject, which is *like* an old man's. It is not old men, but "great Age" which is walking on three feet, with the "leaf already withering." That is, it is the process of aging itself that moves living things and moves as a living thing. "We" do not "get old." Rather "Age" walks on three feet. Not the old men but "strength no greater than a child's dream seen by day wanders." It is the not the old men, but weakened strength that wanders, like a night dream seen by day.

Humans are but shapes put together for the moment, held in a most tenuous unity, no more substantial than leaves. Agents are not agents, but liquids of life flowing into living and dying that gather and dissolve.

Yet these elders, left behind because they were too old to go to Troy, fragile as they are, are convincing in the story they tell of Agamemnon and Menelaus, who set out from Argos with a thousand ships to Troy, because of the way they speak their truth. Their language is set in an oppositional, riddling style, akin to the style of the Delphic Oracle, the voice of divine authority for the ancient Greeks. The Oracle is mimetic of the cosmic laws themselves, bringing them into being and effect as they are spoken.

Oppositions continue in the definition of the scepters on which the old men lean. They are a symbol at once of infirmity and authority. The image of the withering leaf brings into vision not only their decrepitude, but also the thoughtful and vibrant Glaucon and Diomedes exchanging genealogies and armor on Homer's battlefield ("We are as the generation of leaves"). So too do the old men's staves bring to mind the royal scepter held by Agamemnon and Achilles as they speak their opinions in the assembly.

Finally, their reference to the "three footed way" is meant to suggest both the weakness of age and its wisdom. In itself an early riddle proverb, The "three footed way" is a reference to the Sphinx's question to Oedipus: "what walks on four feet in the morning, two in the afternoon, and three at night?" The answer is "man." The old men gain authority and the power of truth as memory (the word for truth in Greek is *aletheia*, or the "absence of forgetfulness") in the allusion to the riddle of the Sphinx. Like the riddle, they contain all three ages in their solution. Like Tiresias the prophet, as well, they are wise because they have experienced all ages. In their evocation of the riddle, they bring the authority of prophecy forward and situate humanity within the Sphinx's riddle.

"Tripleness" itself is evocative of the formulas of oracular language. The familiar statement used to describe the Oracle's authority falls consistently into the same triple pattern. She is the one "who knows the things that are, the things that will be, and the things that were before now": *hos ede ta t'eonta ta t'esomena pro t'eonta.* The chorus, in its own three-footed wisdom holds oracular omniscience:

> I have power to tell of the auspicious command of the expedition, the command of men in authority; for still from the gods am I inspired with persuasive power, my strength in song, by the life that has grown up with me: to tell how …
>
> (Aeschylus, 1979 [Aesch. *Ag.* 104–107])

Sumphutos, to "grow up with," suggests the idea that a person's lifetime is born, grows up, and ages with him. Age here has substance. It grows old itself, and we grow old with it. The "strength of song" gives substance to the insubstantiality and frailty of the aged chorus. The song is breathed into the old men from "godward" (*theothen*). This song will describe an omen from above, interwoven with its interpretation. It is an inspired song, phrased in oracular form. Its "strength" implies the attribution of substance and physical power to words. The omen as it is spoken becomes one with the dramatic action; the pronouncement, one with the fulfillment.

Yet the actual omen which the old men report as being seen, and which the prophet Calchas will interpret, functions as both sign and symbol. This symbol as it is enunciated holds all the action of the play frozen in its cosmic and irrevocable pattern:

> to tell how the two-throned command of the
> Achaeans, of the
> youth of Hellas
> the concordant leadership,
> was sped with avenging spear and arm by the warlike bird of
> omen to the Teucrian land,
> the king of birds appearing to the kings of ships,
> the black eagle and behind it the white one,
> appearing near the palace on the hand in which the spear is brandished,
> in seats conspicuous,
> feeding upon the hare, her womb teeming with young,
> checked from running her final course.
> Sing sorrow, sorrow, but may the good prevail!
> (Aeschylus, 1979 [Aesch. *Ag.* 108–121])

As the Greek expresses it, it appears that even though the expedition against Troy had already been planned, it is the "impetuous omen," *thourios ornis* (literally "bird" here stands for omen), that sends the expedition on its way. The omen is a reflection of the situation on earth, yet it is only when the sign is recognized and interpreted that it can come into being. Speaking the sign in all its implications brings it into human consciousness within the realm of effectiveness. Once it has been recognized, it must be acted upon. In this way it bears similarities to the ratification of any oracle. Human beings look into the sky for signs and the patterns they find indicate *what will be done*. Once the pattern has been imposed and spoken publicly, choice within the limited range of its possibility must inevitably follow. In this sense actions are predetermined.

The phrasing, "the double-throned strength of the Achaian, the together-minded leadership," pairs the two kings, as many are paired in the oracles, and the words "of birds the king, to the kings of ships, one dark, the other white-tailed" exhibits the familiar antithetical correspondences found in many Delphic responses. It is such chiasma and antithesis as this that bring omen and action, sign and what it signifies into unity. The birds are actually flying above the ships they represent. They are as real as the Atreidae (Agamemnon and Menelaus), and so is their action. In the absence of any representation of time expressed through a verb, both sign and what it signifies have equal presence and actuality.

The omen itself is foreboding: "Appearing hard by the hall (or palace) in conspicuous seats (or the place in the sky where omens are to be considered omens) on the spear-wielding side, feeding on the hare, swollen with young, checked from future runnings" (Aeschylus, 1979 [*Ag.* 116–120]). The word "Seats" here connotes the seats of men as well as the omen-place in the sky; "the sky on the spear-wielding side" suggest the Greek leaders in the place of the eagles. The use of the term *laginan gennan*, literally translated as "the race of hares" (of hares used here as an adjectival phrase), portends the utter destruction of future generations. The young are killed in the womb of the "hare-race," as the house of Atreus will continue its killing to utter destruction. In the killing all future births are doomed. Calchas, the prophet, interprets:

> In time does this expedition capture Priam's city,
> and all the abundant herds
> of the people before the walls
> shall Fate violently ravage.
> Only let no envy from the Gods cast in darkness
> struck beforehand, the great bit for Troy's mouth
> that is the army encamped. For in pity holy Artemis is angry
> with the swift hounds of her father
> that sacrifice the wretched hare with all her young before the birth;
> she loathes the feast of the eagles.
> Song sorrow, sorrow, but may the good prevail!

Kindly as the Fair One
to the helpless young of savage lions
and delightful to the breast-loving whelps
of all beasts that roam the wild,
she begs (warns) that these portents be made valid;
favorable, but not faultless are the signs.
(Aeschylus, 1979 [Aesch *Ag.* 126–145])

Like the chorus, Calchas interprets the sign in oppositionally effective language, in words tinged with meaning particular to the past and future fate of the house of Atreus. Also, like the chorus, his language is resonant with obscurity, evident in words such as *keleuthos*, *moira*, and *drosos*. Although they are comprehensible in context, once again they are related to what they represent as cosmic process, taking the place of subject. *Keleuthos* means "path," or "way"; in this place only is the word translated as "expedition." Thus, the literal translation is: "in time this path will seize the city of Troy, and Apportionment (*moira*, which is frequently translated as 'fate') will sack by force the herds belonging to the city, outside the walls."

The interpretation of the sign then is once again phrased in terms of process and eternal law. It is not Agamemnon and Menelaus who will seize the city of Troy, but the path they are on. And it is not they who will sack the city, but the law of apportionment which will take when something has been taken from it. Again, *drosios aeptois maleron leonton* means "the helpless young of fierce lions," but *drosos* means "water," or "pure liquid." Translated literally then, "the helpless liquid of fierce lions" implies an underlying substance that permeates and creates all living creatures. The lions are part of a flowing process of generation, all part of the imagery of blood, which, when it becomes clotted, produces no more young. Thus, part of the obscurity of Calchas' interpretation derives from an ambiguous language that merges the static, bounded object with the process of everlasting changes, underlying substances, and eternal laws. Again, this anticipates Klein's intrapsychic notion of the transformation of primary process into a symbolic, oppositional state.

The language of the portent is both more and less than metaphor. It is a portent seen in the sky announcing the fall of Troy by the violence of the Greek rulers. Yet it is the language of the portent itself that surpasses the reality of the rulers. When Artemis is proclaimed furious at the death of the pregnant hare by the eagles, she is angry only at the imagery of the sign, the prediction. Her function as a divinity is interpreted to mean that the Greeks will ravage Troy. Artemis is actually enraged because she is a protectress of Troy, but in the portent, what provokes her to action is that she sees the young of the hare being killed before birth, together with the pregnant animal. As Calchas says, Artemis is angered at the hare's death. So, it appears that Artemis is angered not just by the event the omen foretells (which is predetermined in its forecasting), but by the sign itself as an in-the-moment reality! Artemis must act because the crime falls within her own specific domain as goddess of childbirth and protectress of the young. And insofar as the goddess incorporates both sides of what she represents, that is, insofar as she is connected with the young both as their protectress and their destroyer, her recompense for such "hare" sacrifice must lead to another sacrifice of the young.

Here, the symbol runs aground in its oppositions. It is submerged in a pattern known from the time of Anaximander, a 6th-century pre-Socratic philosopher:

> The Unlimited is the first-principle of things that are. It is that from which the coming-to-be takes place, and it is that into they return when they perish, by moral necessity, giving satisfaction to one another and making reparation for their injustice, according to the order of time.
>
> (Anaximander, quoted in Wheelwright, 1996, p. 54)

Retribution must be paid for any act committed, in accordance with the order of time. Seasons give way to seasons, and here, in the catastrophe of the deprivation of mother-rights, sacrifice gives way to sacrifice in an enmeshment of gods, humans, and nature. *Tisis*, "retribution" or the "act of vengeance," is expressed through verbal oppositions that are complemented by thematic oppositions. This is also seen in that the word "sacrifice" is used here instead of murder. The "winged hounds" of Artemis' father Zeus are hunters, and as image plays into action, Artemis necessarily demands yet another, the child of Agamemnon himself: Iphigeneia.

As sign and what is signifies become intermingled in this passage, so do ritual and real action within the dramatic context. Agamemnon's act of sacrificing Iphigeneia, his daughter, becomes the ritual that atones for the sacrifice of the hare, a sacrifice that occurs only within the context of the omen and has no base in actual human reality. Humans are swept up in the same equations as are nature and the gods: Thus, confusion between ritual sacrifice that heals and atones for original misbehavior and the actual act of murder that calls for vengeance and then more vengeance in the lives of the family of Atreus is set in motion through the symbol itself and its expression.

Here, image takes on infinite substance, absorbing mere human activity within it. For the eagles are not only Agamemnon and Menelaus. Going back in the ancestry, Zeus himself was the son of Kronos, who ate the rest of his children and wanted to swallow Zeus himself. Zeus' son, Tantalus, served his son Pelops up for the gods to eat. And Pelops, who survived because the gods noticed they were served human flesh and refused to eat, was the father or Atreus, who was served up his own children to eat by his own brother, Thyestes, as punishment for engaging in an adulterous act with his brother's wife. Atreus was the father of Agamemnon. So, the hare is not only Troy, but all banquets of children. The omen describes a process of being in which all the race is held prisoner. Subjects are held in a neither-nor relation. It is the process, the action, that continues without end. The tragic actors are replaceable parts of this process. Yet all this language is still in the starry regions, the space of darkness from which the fiery flash from mountain top to mountain top announcing the end of the Trojan War – carrying the flame of victory is mirrored by Clytemnestra's flame of deceitful persuasion on the inner altars, which will lead to Agamemnon's own destruction (Aeschylus, 1979 [Aesch. *Ag*. 90–97]). There is as yet no will, no possibility for change.

In the chorus as a whole, antithesis speaks authenticity. Common substance is bounded in antithesis. The effort to bound and balance phrases with dualities and antitheses is in itself a way of asserting definitions from the amorphousness of the cosmos in which humans now find themselves.

Now we can see more clearly why the omen, a complex, enveloping symbol set within the dialectic of a narrow, oscillating balance of vengeance and revenge, rings valid for a people who attribute such laws to nature itself. Caught up within its overarching power, they have no power of their own to move beyond it, no sense of what it might mean to break out of its all-encompassing necessity. Yet their oracular speaking of it, in endless repetition, has brought it to the light of day. Chaos and amorphousness are made clear through this order; yet at the same time the order is instantiated through its speaking. Because these figures are creating the very order as it appears, they are neither a part of the eternal cosmic laws nor not a part of them. They are transitional figures, fused, as it were, in a creative process that continues to emanate into destructive patterns because there appears no way out of this oscillation. Cosmic law demands cycles from vengeance to revenge and back again. It all appears hopelessly split, even though it is the ability to verbalize the split in symbolic form that makes a kind of order and consciousness possible.

Here we can see the relevance of Kleinian object-relations theory in specific context. The regnant culture is caught, like the Kleinian infant, in the paranoid-schizoid position, a necessary split if it is to emerge from the amorphous indistinctness of the parent-infant unit, or the matricentric world. The symbol itself is like a Winnicottian transitional phenomenon. The illusion of its concrescence must be kept to keep the connection with Mother as the baby moves into its own creativity and ability to grow. But here, the omen is frighteningly overdetermined, stuck in what Zabriskie calls a "frozen accident" (1997, p. 25): a space of frozen fantasy in which the cultural complex itself cannot move to a new stage because of some giant wounding. Perhaps the wounding here is the very act of agency itself as it moves to a self-awareness that will radically separate it from its earlier way of being. It is as if the ancient Greek world of this fused and talionic family, descended from Zeus, must now make a move to a separate self-awareness and change out of the existing order, to avoid complete annihilation:

> Who shall cast out the brood of curses from the house?
> The race is fastened to destruction.
> (Aeschylus, 1979 [Aesch. *Ag.* 1565–1566])

8.3.2 *Intimations of Will in the* Agamemnon

It appears that there might be a moment of such expression of agency in Agamemnon's choice of evils either to sacrifice his daughter, or the entire Greek army. Vernant and Vidal-Naquet, in the essay "Intimations of the Will in Greek Tragedy" (1988) suggest that we may see the first inklings of will in an often mistranslated stanza referring to Agamemnon when he learns of the omen demanding that he sacrifice his daughter Iphigeneia in return for his going to war against Troy:

> Then the senior prince gave tongue and said,
> "A grievous doom is disobedience,
> and a grievous doom it is
> if I massacre my daughter, the pride of my house,
> polluting with streams of slaughtered maiden's blood
> a father's hands hard by the altar,
> Which of these courses is free from evil?"
> How am I to become a deserter of my ships,
> losing my allies?
> For that they should long
> for a sacrifice to still the winds and for a maiden's blood
> with passion exceeding passion
> is right in the eyes of heaven. May all be for the best!
>
> And when he had put on the yoke-strap of compulsion,
> *his spirit's wind veering to an impious blast,*

> *impure, unholy, from that moment*
> *his mind changed to a temper of utter ruthlessness.* [italics added]
>
> (Aeschylus, 1979 [Aesch. *Ag*. 205–221])

The implication of the last three lines is that even though the act itself is demanded by forces external to Agamemnon ("the yoke-strap of compulsion"), his "spirit's wind" veers in a move akin to a decision that is charged with affect, a possible preliminary stage to the exertion of agency by the will. Yet, in the very act, the same cycle of retribution is stirred all over again, holding the race fastened to contradiction in a repetitive act of vengeance. Indeed, Agamemnon's first move to act in accordance with his own deadly choice is called "impious." Likewise, when he chooses, perhaps out of the hubris that makes him choose to be like the very Asian king he has conquered, to walk on the tapestries of his own house, he once again makes a choice based on the persuasion (this time of his wife in the guise of divine fury, rather than the command of a divine goddess) to pollute the home. He walks on tapestries, called by Clytemnestra "a sea – and who shall dry it up – that breeds a gush of much purple" (Aeschylus, 1979 [Aesch. *Ag*. 958–960]). That is, he enters a river of blood that will lead him, like an ox, to his own murder / sacrifice.

Who can say that this is not an original act of childlike grandiosity that births the infant into the world? He comes having destroyed his mother earth, a maternal, ritual culture, having sacrificed a virgin to keep her from flowering into a fertility that cannot but display mortality in initiating cycles of birth and death. He walks like a hero into his new home, a new agent, and suffers being tangled in a net, thrown into a bath, and stabbed to death by a woman / mother who holds family and ancestral rules close to her heart. Her very act is to her but a sacrifice that brings up flowers in this spring:

> I added a third stroke, a votive offering
> for the Zeus below the earth, the savior of corpses.
> So did he fall and quickly breathed away his life,

> And spouting out a sharp jet of blood
> He struck me with a dark shower of gory dew,
> while I rejoiced no less than the crop rejoices
> in the Zeus-given moisture at the birth of the bud.
> (Aeschylus, 1979 [Aesch. *Ag* 1386–1394])

It is as if the beginnings of agency are themselves impious against the great parental gods. One cannot make a move without the fear of being devoured. What has happened to the original act of ox sacrifice which has no impiety in it, except that in choosing sacred food that one desires is in itself deserving of sacrifice because it is part of the life cycle, is that history has entered the scene. The sacrifice now has a name, is a king, becomes an historical figure living in time, and so cries forth to be an individual. The identification of oppositional laws with oppositional language would work were it still describing a cyclical world of death and rebirth. But narrative has entered, and with it the conflict of the historical figure with the ritual figure. Murder and sacrifice are confused. The eating of children is literalized in the race that now knows its mortality. Devouring and regurgitating are all right in the primitive psyche that knows no distinctions. But when the move has been made into historical narrative, then the nascent self is present. This society already shows that it can recapitulate the symbol in words and can enunciate the opposites of vengeance and revenge, but it cannot move further. Where is the possibility for change and transformation? How does one experience the freedom of being a symbolizing creature?

8.3.3 Cassandra: The Move from Symbol to Symptom

Cassandra opens the possibility of vision and seeing-through. She enters toward the end of the *Agamemnon* with King Agamemnon, on his chariot. The chorus appears unaware of her story as she babbles in barbarian tones. The audience, however, cannot understand her as she calls out the name of her destroyer, Apollo. Having refused to have sex with him, he gave her the gift of prophecy and the curse of never being believed. Here, she acts out her fate, caught in the paradox of being a prophetess of vision who is not believed or understood, caught too in the ambivalence of being loved by the god of light and prophecy, whose name means as well, "destruction." It is the stuttering ambivalence of being caught by heaven and earth, dwelling in this liminal and impossible space that, faced with the crisis of seeing the children of Atreus above the halls of the palace, their guts hanging out, that forces her to take the veil from her face, like a wedding veil, to blurt out the disaster of the house so that it can be understood. She sees at this moment all the acts of vengeance captured in one present horrifying moment of Agamemnon's murder, soon to be her own as well. The vision that encapsulates all the overdeterminations of the past brings her words to clarity and communication with others in her own acceptance of her fate. Here, perchance, is a genuine act of choice, to acknowledge death calmly in the face of one's own imminent death. The crimes of the house are brought to the presence of the stage through her speech and in her murder. All is revealed and named. The wound stands open, pouring free, no longer clotting the earth, because it has been named and heard. It is ambivalence itself that is bared as she calls on Apollo, god of light, as god of destruction. Yet one wonders if the oracular itself has been destroyed in her demise. What happens in the resolution of the paradox?

8.4 Orestes and Melanie Klein

In the *Libation Bearers*, Electra and her brother Orestes meet by the side of their father's tomb, recognize one another, and plot their mother's murder. The language of this play takes the form of hypnotic binding song, or dirge, calling up the spirit of the father's ghost to their aid. Orestes is commanded by Apollo to kill his mother, yet it is clear in his own speech that whether he does so or not, the Furies, ancient and revered goddesses in charge of punishing the killers of kin, and especially of matricides, will visit him with boils and creeping cancers on his skin:

> For as he (Apollo) revealed to mortals the means of mollifying
> malignant powers below the earth, he spoke, naming these
> plagues
> leprous ulcers that mount upon the flesh with cruel fangs,
> eating away its primal nature;
> and a white down sprouting forth upon this infection.
> (Aeschylus, 1979 [Aesch. *Ch.* 279–285])

The nurse who actually breastfed Orestes recognizes him and speeds him on his way to kill Clytemnestra. There is one brief moment, as his own mother bares her breast to him, in which he hesitates, asking his friend Pylades if he should indeed commit this heinous act. But then he drives his sword through her chest.

Clytemnestra has herself anticipated this murder in a dream in which a baby serpent nurses her breast and draws out both blood and milk. The imagery of the good and the bad breast so predominant in Melanie Klein's thinking could not be clearer here. The infant's rage against the mother may well arise from a sense that it will be devoured, all the more powerful if the mother, identified with mother earth, has become a killer of males in response to a world that has rejected her. Orestes' need for revenge stems from his own sense of persecution, here literally realized in the play through his exile. His own projected anger against Clytemnestra then comes back to haunt him in the guise of a punishing superego, here understood in the form of part objects not yet internalized, played by the parent gods Apollo, the Furies, Zeus, and Athena.

Klein, in a little-known, posthumously published essay on the *Oresteia* (1940/1963), suggests that Orestes moves beyond the paranoid-schizoid state evident in the earlier plays to a place of guilt. Orestes may feel that he has lost his mother through his own "greedy and destructive impulses" (p. 313). The recognition of his simultaneous love and hate for Clytemnestra, perhaps symbolized in the breast from which he, as a baby serpent, draws both milk and blood, provokes "mourning and pining" for the lost object, as well as guilt stemming from his sense of responsibility for destroying that object. For Klein, guilt and depression are the results of coming to terms with our own aggressive impulses. In the *Oresteia*, Orestes can be seen as a young man who is greedy to attain the kingdom of his father and cannot bear it that his mother is occupying it with a lover. Symbolically, Orestes may stand for the male libido that must free itself from mother earth to gain his own kingdom, especially when the race appears to be fastened to destruction and the never-ending cycle of vengeance and revenge.

Guilt leads to compassion and the desire to make reparation. For Klein, Orestes is the perfect representation of the self being born. She says:

> In my view he shows the mental state which I take to be characteristic of the transition between the paranoid-schizoid and the depressive position, a stage when guilt is essentially experienced as persecution. When the depressive position is reached and worked through – which is symbolized in the Trilogy by Orestes' changed demeanor at the Areopagus – guilt becomes predominant and persecution diminishes.
>
> (1940/1963, p. 286)

Klein states that Athena, in the *Eumenides*, represents the balance of the paranoid-schizoid position, as Zeus represents good, mild father, who can judge fairly. The Furies and Apollo, however, represent the primitive impulses. Apollo holds rage and aggression against the woman because she is fertile, cyclical, and independent, as seen by his idealization of the armored, virginal Athena, the father's daughter, his hatred of the older female Furies, his non-sympathy with Clytemnestra as mother in claiming the male as sole parent, and his earlier cruelty to Cassandra.

Klein's attempt to understand the *Oresteia* goes some way to understanding what is one of the most difficult transformations in all of Greek tragedy: the transformation of the dread Furies in charge of matricides into the Eumenides, good spirits of birth and marriage. But, ultimately, her argument does not see the constrictions to the possibility of self-birth for Orestes, which is primarily revealed through the change in the way language is used in the *Eumenides*, as well as through the authority of Apollo over Orestes, and Orestes' ultimate inability to escape the Furies.

In this final play of the trilogy, Apollo appears in his role as healer to break this magic spell, or *thelkterion*, and he says as much to Orestes in words that recall the magic means at play in the *Agamemnon*:

> Do not grow weary as you struggle to cope with this
> ordeal; but go to the city of Pallas
> and sit there, taking her ancient image in your arms.
> and there shall we have judges of your cause, and words
> to charm them, and shall discover means
> to release you forever from this distress;
> for it was I who persuaded you to slay your mother.
> (Aeschylus, 1979 [Asch. *Eum*. 78–84])

The word *thelkterion* means "spell" or "charm." It is a force that works irrationally to possess the mind. Used as a word in witchcraft, it is also often associated with divine influence in respect to the spellbinding power of poetry and rhetoric in 5th-century Athens (Romilly, 1975). It is in this later sense that Apollo uses it. The words he persuades with will no longer be those of witchcraft and spell, but rather those of the legal rhetoric of the Athenian court. These will serve as the means to transformation, taking over from the authority of oracles and signs. The Delphic Oracle was accustomed to receiving prayers asking for a "release from pains (*apallangē ponōn*)." Apollo will do this by releasing minds from the "binding song" of the Oracle itself.

Athena, too, plays her part in tethering the magically effective to the rules of the new political order and the scales of Zeus. When the chorus tell her that Orestes killed his mother, and Athena asks if there was no other force driving his wrath, they refuse to consider that such possibility might exist. Nothing, they say, is of such consequence, or weighs so heavy in the scales as matricide. Athena will not let them get away with simply stating that this unwritten law is stronger than all argument. She states that only half of the case has been heard. The chorus says that Orestes refused to swear an oath, and again rests its judgment on the effective power of the spoken phrase. But Athena overrules the chorus, saying no longer is the oath to have its irredeemable power. It is rather to be joined to the judgments men make through rational discourse. The formerly uncontrollable force that, for example, could send a curse elsewhere simply by its evocation in words is now bereft of its archaic magic in that it can be harnessed to human reason.

The possibility that a formerly frozen symbolic system, frozen in so far as it is part of a cultural unconscious, can, with the use of reason, become open to action based on human choice as it begins to engage humans as conscious agents is both freeing and imprisoning. The move from magical language to legal language engages magical language to invoke legal persuasion. In this way, we could say from a psychotherapeutic stance that it engages the language of unconscious subliminal process to transform consciousness but, in so doing, it loses track of a profound psychic level of functioning that connects human beings to other forms of life, as well as to their own biological and psychological foundations, to exalt the power of rational and legal discourse over all.

In the dialogue between the Furies and Orestes, as well as between the Furies and Apollo, the premises are refuted specifically point for point. Orestes asserts that his father will send him protection from his grave. The Furies respond directly, demanding to know how he would ask for help from the dead, since he killed his mother. Orestes responds that there are two counts against her: she killed a man, and that man was his father. Again, the Furies respond by pointing out that Clytemnestra did not kill a blood relative, whereas Orestes did.

Orestes then turns his defense over to Apollo, who justifies his own command to Orestes to kill Clytemnestra by saying that it came from a higher authority, namely Zeus. The chorus demands to know how Zeus can ordain such a *chrēsmos*, the technical word for a command or an oracle, when Zeus himself dishonored his own father. Apollo answers with legal hairsplitting, using the same argument that has been the chorus' mainstay throughout the trilogy: Zeus bound his father. For the Furies, binding is not the same as killing. Blood cannot be recalled.

Three things have happened here that bring the point-by-point defense into question. First, Apollo is not arguing justice in the cosmic moral sense; he is arguing a legal point. Apollo's world is that of the law court, implying that the human world does not need to bother with cosmic and unwritten law. Second, Apollo is justifying his case with the use of a very particular myth, chosen to meet the demands of the particular accusation. It is being consciously used at this point in the play to win an argument. Apollo is using a shaky precedent to prove his case.

Apollo's third and victorious moment comes when he makes use of new, presumably scientific knowledge in asserting that Orestes is not actually a blood relative of his mother, and therefore the Furies cannot hold him guilty. Apollo's confirming proof for this is Athena herself, who needed no mother to be born. Athena is a rare case. Nevertheless, she is here, as *tekmerion*, or "evidence." It is difficult to believe that in making this the pivotal moment of Apollo's argument Aeschylus was not casting an ironic and perhaps not wholly approving eye on the legal machinations available to the Athenian court.

The Furies are not in the least convinced by the new logic. Athena only succeeds in persuading them when she fights their repetitive curses with repetitive affirmations that they will be transformed. In the course of her persuasion, she uses a verbal transformation, changing the alpha-privative triple curse into a triple blessing, beginning not with "*a*" but with "*eu*":

> *toiauth' helesthai soi parestin ex emou*
> *eu drosan, eu pasxousin, eu timomenen*
> *choras metaschei tesde theophilestates*
> (Aesch. *Eum.* 867–869)

> Such is the good choice I offer you:
> to do good and receive good, and in goodly honor
> to have a portion in this land most dear to the gods.
> (Aeschylus, 1979)

This verbal transformation is closely bound to the Furies' transformation from goddesses upholding the rights of murdered kin into goddesses of marriage and childbirth. And it is not insignificant that Athena, just before they are convinced and transformed, asks them to honor the *peithous sebas glossēs emēs meiligma kai thelktērion*: "Persuasion's majesty/ The power to charm and soothe that sits upon my tongue" (Aeschylus, 1979 [Aesch. *Eum.* 885–886]). *Thelkterion* has here indeed become a new "charm," this time of rhetorical words. Athena herself thanks Persuasion, who *epopa*, "watches over," her voice and tongue (the same verb so often used of the all-seeing ability of the gods and the Pythia).

For Klein, true depression and the capacity for reparation and forgiveness shine through the pageantry at the end of the *Eumenides*, as Athena persuades the Furies to change their mind and sends them beneath the Areopagus. There is in fact a sense in which one can see that the Furies are persuaded through mirroring and empathy. Athena not only uses the language of magical persuasion that they are familiar with to persuade them, but she wears on her aegis the snake-headed Medusa that must remind them of themselves.

As helpful as Klein is in her analysis, there is a strong sense in this last play that she has been duped – that there is a liminal stage between pre-symbolic and symbolic process that is as absent in this early Greek solution to finding agency as it is in Freud and Klein. There seems to be no satisfactory channel for transition from symbolic oppositions to a growth that can produce an integrated or whole self.

There is a strong hint of this in the staging of the *Eumenides* as well. It appears that intermediaries between gods and men, such as symbols, omens, or signs, are no longer needed. Gods present themselves on stage as if they are simply larger mortals with more authority, leaving us wondering whether there are any more gods out there beyond mortals or any mystery left at all. When the gods present themselves on stage and the charms of persuasion are open to men to control, there is no longer any place for the Oracle, either. The mysteries of the cosmos can now be solved by the particular law addressing itself to the particular situation.

Something huge has been lost if there is no answer to the case that can satisfy both sides of the equation. Orestes could have been judged guilty of murdering his mother, yet still be given a light sentence judging the merits of his particular case. If the trial had been composed by Aeschylus in this way, then the container of the mother both as individual mother and as an earth mother embodying ritual culture and unwritten law would stay intact, and still hold promise for the birth of the transitional process in human development that leads to the recognition of the individual unit of the baby apart from its mother, or the nascent self, integrated with its community and its own interiority.

Acknowledging the birth of the symbolic subject would have allowed the ancient Greek audience to affirm the balances, oppositions, and riddles inherent in ancient Greek thinking. But here, as we have seen, in order to acquit Orestes, one side of the case, namely that the mother is indeed a blood relation to her son, which Aeschylus must have understood and certainly assumes in all his other plays, has been summarily dismissed. (Because Aeschylus was himself an initiate of the Eleusinian Mysteries, based on the sacrality of Demeter and Persephone, mother and daughter, it is convincing to me that one of the messages he was giving the Athenians in the *Eumenides* was that it was imperative to preserve a strong sense of connection with the collective and with the matricentric world.)

This rejection and overpowering of cosmic laws cannot help but be catastrophic. For where there is no more tolerance for ambiguity and spells no longer hold any authenticity, mysteries themselves tend to disappear. Although this may satisfy our rational egos, it does not satisfy the human spirit that wishes to be interconnected with gods, nature, and community.

Athena, herself, empathic and convincing as she may be to the Furies, stands for the immortality of the state, human reason, and not female fertility. She is an armored female, quite antithetical to a more frequent ancient Greek image of females as leaking jars, hysterical erotic creatures (the Danaids) who cannot contain their evils (Pandora). Their evils turn out to be that they leak children, proving the mere mortality of human beings.

Further, Athena's magic has been turned to official use. It has become mere rhetoric to serve the new city-state. The language of Apollo is the expository language of the lawcourt, setting precedents through particulars. Orestes is not acquitted because he might have a legitimate reason to kill his mother. He is acquitted because his only blood parent turns out to be his father. Apollo, with Athena setting precedent, declares that Clytemnestra was never Orestes' mother, but only a basket that held his father's seed. Apollo's claim is that Orestes is not her blood kin. Here, the riddle is not solved, but one side of the paradox/riddle is simply eliminated. The riddling language of the *Agamemnon*, along with the binding chant of the *Libation Bearers*, is thrown out together with the symbolic language that holds the paradoxes.

The result is that women go underground, the repressed unconscious is born, holding the seeds of destruction that require an armored ego to resist them. Proof of this is that Orestes, though acquitted legally, is nevertheless driven insane by the Furies, and shows up as mad in all the succeeding Greek tragedies of Sophocles and Euripides (see Dobson, "Why Does Orestes Stay Mad?" in *Psychology and the Classics* (2018) De Gruyter Press).

Klein would agree that there can be no depression or reparation without unifying of splits in the individual. But the last of Aeschylus' plays in this trilogy celebrates the instigation of the city-state and the formation of a brittle, vulnerable ego. It is an ego with which we are all too familiar today. It displays a false self, highly rational and political, hiding beneath it a world of suffering and mother absence.

References

Aeschylus (1979). *The Oresteia* (H. Lloyd Jones, trans.). Berkeley, CA.: University of California Press.

Aristotle (1983). *Poetics*. In H.G. Apostle and L.P. Gerson (trans.), *Aristotle: Selected Works*. Grinnell, IA: Peripatetic Press, pp. 645–681.

Campbell, J. (ed.) (1971). *The Portable Jung* (R.F.C. Hull, trans.). New York: Penguin Books.

Dobson, M. (2018). Why does Orestes stay mad? In J. Lauwers, H. Schwall, J. Opsomer (eds.), *Psychology and the Classics: A Dialogue of Disciplines*. Berlin: De Gruyter, pp. 158–170.

Harrison, J.E. (1962a). *Epilegomena to the Study of Greek Religion and Themis: A Study of the Social Origins of Greek Religion.* New York: University Books.

Klein, M. (1963). Some reflections on Aeschylus' *Oresteia.* In *Envy and Gratitude and other Works*. New York: Free Press, pp. 275–299. (Original work published in 1940.)

Onians, R.B. (1951). *The Origins of European Thought* (2nd ed.). Cambridge, UK: Cambridge University Press.

Padel, R. (1992). *In and out of the Greek Mind: Greek Images of the Tragic Self.* Princeton, NJ: Princeton University Press.

Romilly, J. (1975). *Magic and Rhetoric in Ancient Greece.* Cambridge, MA: Harvard University Press.

Vernant, J.P. and Vidal-Naquet, P. (1988). Intimations of the will in Greek tragedy. In *Myth and Tragedy in Ancient Greece.* New York: Urzone, pp. 49–84.

Wheelwright, P. (ed.) (1966). *The Presocratics.* New York: Odyssey Press.

Zabriskie, B. (1997). Thawing the "frozen accidents": The archetypal view in countertransference. *Journal of Analytical Psychology*, 42: 25–40.

Chapter 9

Heroic Catastrophes and Matricentric Coherences

9.1 Introduction

According to Sophocles in *Oedipus Colonus*, the Furies, once rageful representatives of the abandoned mother world, take on a sacred habitat in Colonus, just outside of Athens, a green and leafy grove where pollution must not enter. Now known as Eumenides, goddesses most revered, they and their rites are safely contained outside city boundaries. The town of Eleusis, sacred ground of Demeter and the *kore*, or "maiden" Persephone, opens itself to the Greek populace once a year for a grand viewing of the sacred agricultural mysteries represented through the myth of a mother and daughter. Through this celebration, supplicants become initiates, blessed with the possibility of immortal life. It is significant that these goddesses, powerful representatives and functionaries of earlier matricentric beliefs, are now overseen by a male priesthood. Although revered by the Athenians and other Greeks, they are encoded into civilized, politicized rituals that pose no threat to the patriarchal governance of Athens. Rather, they are co-opted into it and enhance it at a safe distance (cf. Foley, 1994; Downing, 1994).

Within the city walls, Pericles builds his Parthenon, manages the wealth of what comes to be called an empire, and the Athenians become known as the city of democracy, law, and philosophy. Thucydides, the first political scientist, denigrates the compositions of Homer and Herodotus, claiming that they are filled with poetic exaggeration and stories to delight for the moment. In his own work, Thucydides banishes oracles from his

DOI: 10.4324/9781003340751-11

history, calling them superstitious, and claiming to see things as they really are:

> The absence of romance in my history will, I fear, detract somewhat from its interest; but if it be judged useful by those inquirers who desire an exact knowledge of the past as an aid to the interpretation of the future, which in the course of human things must resemble if it does not reflect it, I shall be content. In fine, I have written my work, not as an essay which is to win the applause of the moment, but as a possession for all time.
>
> (Thucydides, 1951, *The Peloponnesian War*, ed. and trans. J.H. Finley, Jr. [*Thuc.* Bk. I, paras. 23–24])

Thucydides understands human nature as expressed through state politics to be driven by "fear," "honor," and "self interest" (p. 44). He addresses women only once, through the funeral oration of Pericles, who says that the greatest glory "is hers who is least talked of among the men whether for good or for bad" (p.109).

Plato, in the 4th century, recalls the great Socrates, who engages in dialectic to find truth. In his *Republic*, Plato recounts the workings of the perfect city, casting out myth, Homer, and the gods, because they do not teach virtue, but instead revel in myths that delight in immoral tales of the gods. Plato redefines the psyche to mirror the state, carefully hierarchized, exalting reason above emotion and internalizing the will. This kind of self-organization is crucial, according to Plato, for the development of ideal citizens.

But the dramatists tell a different story. Sophocles and Euripides turn for their subject matter to the ancient heroic legends of Thebes, an outlying city that bears a reputation for civil wars and incest. Here, the underbelly of rationality thrives. Here, unconscious forces come back to haunt Oedipus in the guise of the Sphinx and his mother. Here, Dionysus destroys Thebes and its king, Pentheus, by driving his mother Agave, along with the rest of the Theban women, into Dionysian frenzy. Agave rips

Pentheus apart like an animal and brings his head back to the city on her thyrsus, believing it to be a lion she has slain.

From a political perspective, one could say that the dramatists delighted in giving negative press to Thebes, a city that Athens prided herself on surpassing in her own rationality and capacity for compassion. Yet mythically and psychologically, the Athenian dramatists after Aeschylus wrote for Athenians, not for Thebans. Their stories, therefore, could only evoke the chaotic emotions and sense of fatedness at the hands of the gods that the new beliefs in rationality and agency had tried to suppress and control, but which simmered with a fervor that split not only psyches but cities, as democrats and aristocrats joined in conflicts that brought about their own downfall through internal dissension, over and over again.

The primary victim repressed in the name of reason and agency was the sacred, imaginal world of the Homeric and archaic Greeks. This world had previously peopled the Greek air and landscape with demons, gods, and omens. It was now radically severed, as are limbs from a body. To function in the democracy, human beings needed to become cohesive and coherent self-agents. The structure of the mind must become compartmentalized and artful. Gods, demons, and women, who, like the Danaids and Pandora, were symbolically identified with vessels that leak, needed to be banished in the name of containing emotions and of invoking individual will and the possibility for choice. Oracles and signs fell under suspicion as expressing only the political manipulations of priests and prophets who vied for power with city leaders. This split in consciousness began a movement in western civilization that eventually necessitated the very invention of modern psychology, which tried to uncover, to discover behind the armored ego embodied by Athena, the divine, non-rational forces the Greeks sent down to the underworld and out from their city boundaries.

Perhaps this split in consciousness was necessary for our greatest human achievement – self-awareness and the interiorization of consciousness, which allow us to engage in reasoned activity in the illusion, at least, that we can separate ourselves as authoritative subjects in the invocation of our distinction from nature, community, and the divine. But the move to reason and against myth appears for our western ancestors to have been accompanied by, if not invented by, the patriarchy, and to have privileged the ego as a presence disconnected from others and the ritual world, as well as from the emotional body. The ego was allowed a reality no longer accorded to the multiple forces of nature and divinities. It lived outside the world of myths, consciously and intentionally attempting to conform the world to its gaze. The need to do this emanated from a strongly held belief in ancient psychology that "the psyche takes on the form of what it intends" (Riker, 1997, p. 33).

This chapter explores some of the devastations of this move. It also explores an ancient Greek text that celebrates relations among women, *The Homeric Hymn to Demeter*, in which an intersubjective reality appears that evokes the possibility for an integrity of mind and soul quite different from the heroic or ego model that we in the west, so encouraged by 5th-century Athens and its descendants, have tended to follow. The intersubjective moments of this Hymn stay in the imaginal, honoring multiplicity and soul without fearing madness or loss of control. They lend ballast to what contemporary feminist and archetypal psychologists are advocating as spiritually therapeutic journeys whose criteria for help embrace multiplicity in wholeness. These psychologists put the notion of self as radically distinct from other into question as a model for health, and demand the presence of intersubjectivity and the imaginal as the only possibility for coming to an integrated consciousness with self and world (cf. Sullivan, 1940; Stolorow, Brandschaft and Atwood, 1987, 1994).

9.2 Brittle Heroes

Although Aeschylus' Orestes comes into his own as a state-pardoned mother killer, one tragic hero after another in Greek drama tries to maintain the integrity of his civic values and fails, or worse, goes mad, because of the continuing pull of a mother world that, like Medusa, shows its teeth in a fatal smile evoked by the hero's repressed desire. In Euripides' *Hippolytus* (428 BCE) Hippolytus, son of Theseus, is brought down by Aphrodite, goddess of love and fertility, because of his solitary worship of Artemis, the virgin huntress. Hippolytus demands a singular purity and virginity for himself, one that refuses to let women or sexuality touch him (see Devereux, 1985; Slater, 1968). Creon, in Sophocles' *Antigone* (441 BCE), negates the unwritten laws of custom and nature associated with family in refusing to let Antigone bury the brother who attacked his own city. Political and natural law storm together as Creon buries Antigone alive and calls his son, engaged to Antigone, a "woman" for having feelings. Haemon says to Creon that he would "rule a desert beautifully alone" (Sophocles I, 1973, E. Wyckoff trans. [Soph. *Ant.* 739]), emphasizing the extent of Creon's isolation from the community. Creon proves a removed and rigid ruler, incapable of honoring natural or ritual laws as he attempts to keep his state, and his head together.

Euripides' *Bacchae* (406 BCE) has as its subject Dionysus, god of tragedy himself, as well as god of all the liquids of life, of multiplicity and metamorphosis. The *Bacchae* is an immensely complex work, which starkly exhibits the fate of a political, presumably rational, hero, Pentheus, fighting against a God who celebrates the natural and non-rational. Much of the discussion about the *Bacchae*, especially in the wake of Nietzsche's *Birth of Tragedy*, focuses on the mental catastrophe that repression of the natural can bring (cf. Segal 1981, 1986).

Social psychological studies of 5th-century Athens tried to diagnose the particular catastrophes faced by tragic heroes. Slater (1968), in a largely Freudian treatise, finds the unremitting narcissism of Greek males to be deeply tied into their desperate need to be affirmed by mothers who could be nothing but ambivalent, given their devalued position in the *polis*. At the same time, the exclusiveness of the mother-son relation during the first four years of life brought the son to identify deeply with his mother, which left him also feeling ambivalent: "The rejection of and dependence upon women mirror the mother's own ambivalence" (p.44). For Gouldner (1965), "The Greeks were deeply concerned about their capacity to go murderously berserk" (p. 109), and their constant concern with moderation, or keeping within limits, showed the "insatiability of their (narcissistic) needs" (p. 69). C. Fred Alford (1992) stresses that sacrifice itself, the essence of the Dionysian ritual, in which one destroys and digests the beloved object, marks the epitome of ambivalence or the split object relation (pp. 61–62; cf. Segal, 1982, pp. 67–68). Bennett Simon (1978) concerns himself with the "incipient psychosis of every tragic hero" (p. 89).

All of these social psychological and psychoanalytic analyses of the ancient Greek tragic hero complement the interpretation here that the recently formed rigid and brittle ego of the Greek male was deeply tied to the structure of the Greek *polis*, which was seeking boundaries to contain and foster humans with a sense of reason, agency, and choice as part of a civic democracy. This so-called democratic polis as we have begun to see, pushed nature, women, and emotion to its edges and to the edges of consciousness, and this repression and expulsion brought both the women of tragedy and the mother world as introjected into the male psyche back to haunt it. It was the very rigidity of these boundaries, seen as essential to the formation of a cohesive (male) self who could function as an independent political being, that brought on the madness of Pentheus and of many others like him (cf. Dodds, 1951; Segal, 1986). It is worth considering two plays in some detail, Euripides' *Bacchae* and Sophocles' *Oedipus Tyrannos*, for the insight they can give into the psychological splitting suffered by the ancient Greek tragic hero.

Euripides' *Bacchae*. Euripides' *Bacchae* (trans. 1974) pits two male cousins against each other, one who believes himself to be a god (Dionysus), and one who is the ruler of Thebes (Pentheus). In their hubristic arrogance, neither is willing to recognize the other's realm of power. Dionysus, then, becomes in this play a hero who suffers the same anthropomorphic and patriarchal rigidities as does his mortal cousin. Dionysus lost his mother Semele to his father Zeus' lightning bolt before he was born and so is motherless with a distant father. Pentheus' mother, Agave, is conspicuous for her hatred of males, at least in her Bacchic trance. Both protagonist and antagonist, therefore, are without mothers and have distant or ambivalent fathers.

Not only does Pentheus show his response to mother abandonment on a family and ritual level by feeling persecuted by Dionysus for his having cast a spell on the women of his city; he is also outraged that his grandfather and the respective prophet of the city, Tieresias, are themselves off to worship the god. Without justification, Pentheus questions their loyalty and trustworthiness. He is unwilling to stand up for his own family or to be close to his near relatives. He is isolated from family, religion, and nature. He repudiates all nurture from others. He is clearly in fear of losing his own independence and power to his cousin. He is envious and jealous, and quick to counterattack what he perceives is an attack on himself from the prophet. He is extra moralistic in his judgment of his aunt and of Dionysus. We see his pristine moralism again when Dionysus tells him that every Eastern land dances his mysteries. "No doubt," Pentheus replies, "their moral standards fall far below ours" (Euripides, 1954, P. Vellacott, trans. [Eur. *Bacch*, 483]).

It is clear from Pentheus' description of the women on the mountain side not only that he feels they are persecuting him, but that he deeply desires his "mother's arms" (Euripides, 1954 [Eur. *Bacch*, 969]), a desire that has turned sexual in its infantile longing. As Pentheus and Dionysus go off to see the Bacchantes, the following dialogue twists us into its double message:

D. I will bring you safely to the place. Another will conduct you back.
P. My mother, yes?
D. A sight for all to witness.
P. To this end I go.
D: You will return borne high
P: Royal magnificence!
D: In my own mother's arms.
P: You insist that I be spoiled.
D: One of a kind spoiling.
P: Yet I win what I deserve.

(Euripides 1954 [Eur. *Bacch*. 965–970])

The "royal magnificence" in which Pentheus will be "borne" stands at once for his sense of entitlement to nourishment and his unconscious fear of decapitation, that is, the impotency of falling into the chaos of mother desire, which is equivalent for him to loss of reason. In Kleinian terms, Pentheus desperately fears being devoured by his own greedy need for a nourishment, and his persecutory reactions to this need are projected onto the Bacchic women. The savage rage of these women seems a corresponding response to Pentheus' own aggression in the face of maternal deprivation. In this situation all he can do is to withdraw from his overpowering emotions into a place of schizoid untouchability. There is no way, given his ambivalence regarding the female world and all it represents, that Pentheus can be anything but split. There is no possibility for remorse or reparation.

Dionysus, who lures this victim to the kill by dressing him in women's clothing and making him see "two Thebes, a double sun" (Eur., 1954, p. 225), appears in the play as a female-identified male named "Bromius" or "Thunderer." Pentheus is gradually drawn by Bromius into the Dionysian ritual. When Dionysus escapes the chains Pentheus has put on him and tricks Pentheus into tying up a bull, thinking it is he, when he has him fighting with phantoms, thinking his own palace is burning down and destroying his own stables, then we can see that symbols are breaking down into primary process formulations and that Pentheus has become fragmented and delusional. If the curly-locked, effeminate Bromius is himself part of Pentheus' delusion, then Pentheus displays a female identification in his splitting away from his male state that we might say moves him toward a fused identification with his mother, exactly what he most deeply and unconsciously desires and fears. Dionysus/Bromius himself appears a split figure: in one manifestation the orgiastic shape-transforming nature god, originary son of mother earth, and in another the son of the patriarchy, who rules women and sees fit to drive them insane for rejecting his worship (for more on the Bacchantes, see Euripides' *Bacchae*, ed. E.R. Dodds, 1974).

A ritual understanding of the action of this tragedy shows that Pentheus is a substitute victim for the Dionysian ritual of *sparagmos* itself. He is the living sacrifice that will presumably be eaten in a sacred communion with nature so that crops will come again and the grapes will burgeon. But what was a natural ritual in the world of the tribe as Harrison explains it has here become a perversion because, once again, it takes place in historical time. That is, it is all well and good for a priestess to sacrifice an animal victim with whom the tribe feels that it shares a totemic identity, but for mother to decapitate an identified king of a 5th-century Greek polis under the illusion that he is a lion will not do.

Euripides' *Bacchae* was produced posthumously in Macedonia, after the author had exiled himself voluntarily from Athens. Insofar as this play is celebratory of Dionysus (who, once again, is a God of tragedy himself), Euripides appears to be suggesting that tragedy itself, as a mode of holding and expressing the splits in the Athenian psyche, is itself at an end. This play was delivered at the very end of Athenian democracy, after Athens had fallen to the Spartans. It was the last of the great tragedies.

Sophocles' *Oedipus the King*. Perhaps because Sophocles himself was a member of a mystery religion and a priest of Asclepius, he was able to express at its fullest and most telling the conflict of an overly rational patriarchy attempting to escape the enmeshment of the matricentric world. He struggled with the story of Oedipus for his entire life, which spanned the 5th century. Sophocles' *Antigone*, although dealing with the struggles of Antigone, Oedipus' daughter, was composed first. The *Oedipus Tyrannos* (*Oedipus the King*) was produced in Sophocles' middle age. Sophocles then continued the story almost as if it were a kind of autobiography into his and Oedipus' old age, in the *Oedipus Coloneus*. (*Oedipus at Colonus*) (406 BCE) probably produced in the same year as Euripides' *Bacchae*.

In *Oedipus Tyrannos*, King Oedipus has become the savior of Thebes because he has solved the riddle of the Sphinx, a female monster who puts potential rulers of the city to the test and kills them if they cannot answer her correctly. Her riddle, "what walks on four feet in the morning, two in the noon, and three at night," the answer to which is "man", is answered by Oedipus, who is lame. He is a "man" who has not from birth ever walked on two feet. Perhaps it is this handicap that has given him the power of observation period Oedipus is a wise and intelligent ruler, who feels deeply for his fellow citizens, and yet he remains unaware of the answers to riddles he constantly speaks that could give him the answer to the question of who he really is as a man: "My pitiable children ... I know well that you all are sick, yet being sick, I know there is not one of you who is equally as sick as I myself" (Sophocles 1, 1973, D. Grene, trans. [Soph. *OT* 60–61]). Sophocles often works with puns, and the words meaning "I know well" in Greek, "*eu gar* (*oid hoti*)" sound not unlike the beginning of his name (Oi-di)pous, indeed the way the above lines are structured poetically in Greek show the synonymy and identification of the sickness of Oedipus and his community:

> *noseite pantes, kai nosountes, hos egō.*
> *Ouk estin humōn ostis ex isou nosei.*
> (Soph. *O.T.* 60–61)

Oedipus is a man who is so intent on searching out the truth with his brilliant mind that he cannot see the crime that he has committed; he cannot hear the irony of the Oracle's words to seek a solution for troubles that "lie at our feet" (Sophocles, 1973 [Soph. *O.T.* 67]). His name means "swollen foot," and was received from the swelling produced by the spikes which were pounded through his feet when he was exposed on Mt. Cithaeron as an infant and left to die, after his father had received the oracle that Oedipus would destroy Thebes. Oedipus' name is close to the word *oida*, which means "I know," so that we know he is both surefooted in his thinking, and also always off the mark: "I have gone many ways 'wandering' in thought" ([Soph. *O.T.* 67]).

Oedipus was rescued by a shepherd, who took him to the childless King and Queen of Corinth, to raise as their own. Called a bastard (*nothos*) at a dinner party by a drunken guest, Oedipus was distressed enough to set off for Delphi – a long journey, especially for a man who limped – and was told when he asked who he was that he would kill his father and marry his mother. Leaving Corinth in a great hurry so as to avoid his fate, Oedipus met an older man in a carriage on the crossroads who, being very much of the same impatient temper as Oedipus, wouldn't let him pass, so Oedipus killed him (his father). He then solved the riddle of the Sphinx and became king of Thebes, marrying its widow, who was old enough to be his mother, and who indeed was his mother.

What comes clear in a reading of the drama through its symbols and story is that Oedipus was, like Pentheus and Dionysus, in all important respects orphaned from his mother and the matricentric world. He used his remarkable intelligence to guide him through the world at the expense of the intuition that lay repressed in the inchoate maternal darkness that was for him a source of great ambivalence. His brightness of vision obscured the evidence that he was sleeping with his mother, which becomes clearer and clearer through the play as he becomes more and more obtuse to this recognition.

Oedipus, while searching for the light, is simultaneously knowingly and unknowingly going back into the darkness of his mother's womb, bearing children who are his sisters and brothers, stopping the flow of time, and bringing plague and famine to the land, because his *hamartia* ("missing the mark," or "intellectual error," often translated "tragic flaw") is in fact not only his anger or "hubris," as is frequently interpreted, but his sharp-sighted intellect. Oedipus can solve the generic riddle, "man," but does not know himself as a human being. His returning to the darkness of his mother's womb is a longing to be with the mother he never had, and so to be in a state of oceanic bliss where no ego is yet born. It is a compensation for his brilliance, a light matched by an equal darkness. When he blinds himself with his wife/mother's brooches by stabbing them into his eyes, he reverses and displaces the sex act, going once more back into the same darkness as he did before, his own eyes now acting as a dark womb, the pins of the brooches his own phallus turned against himself as a kind of self-persecution that will force the pollution to explode out of him and consequently save the city.

At least in the *Oedipus Tyrannos*, the tragedy of Oedipus is that he strove too much for the light, the logical answers, the reasoned response. He killed the female sphinx and ran from a mother who was not his mother in order to avoid pollution, but ended up in the midst of incest. The sense of being without a mother evoked his need and his deep sense of abandonment, which in turn drew him into a sexual attachment with her that destroyed him.

Yet, if one looks at early myths of the ancient Mediterranean, they all tell stories of the mother goddess and her son consort. The incestuous act of sleeping with the son is the only way to produce offspring to populate the cosmos. This happens because mothers always come first, sons after, and mothers appear not to have or to need husbands until the sex act is understood as that which produces children. It is the ritual act of mother sleeping with son that births the world. If this is the case, we are left asking the question why is incest suddenly such a pollution in the *Oedipus Tyrannos*? The answer may be that Oedipus has entered historical, political time, and that in such a realm, a mother who sleeps with her son stops linear time. No children will be born who are not of the same generation as the father, and so related to him as sister and brother. Oedipus cannot birth descendants. This is why infants die and crops cannot grow. In addition, the extent of family fusion and confusion in this game of incest allows for no distinction, no moving out into the polis. Family still reigns supreme. Psychologically, this is equivalent to the fused state of primary process and pre-symbolic life, where there is no possibility for transitional space to occur such that one can move into a self-other relation. Oedipus Tyrannos could never comprehend metaphor; he'd rather function as one entirely separate, rigid, and autonomously defensive. He was unable to authenticate himself except by defending himself through the light of his intellect, thus denying the world of the mother. Although some think that his putting out his eyes is an extraordinary expression of guilt and remorse in the face of an inevitable fate, it is clear that it is also a desperate move to gain rational control:

> It was Apollo, friends, Apollo,
> that brought this bitter bitterness, my sorrows to completion.
> But the hand that struck me
> was none but my own.
>
> (Sophocles, 1973 [Soph. *O.T.* 1467–71])

To such ends has this path to reason and autonomy found its way!

9.3 Matricentric Coherences and Relational Being: The Homeric Hymn to Demeter

As we have seen, the Greek patriarchal voice cried out for ways to become self-ruling in a world felt as dangerously fluid and chaotic. Tragedy and epic both have shown us vulnerable heroes, reeling with frequent and sudden polytheistic disruptions that affect both inner and outer nature. In contrast, the Eleusinian mysteries, which celebrate the mother-daughter bond, present a radical alternative to the abrupt separation from the matricentric world that Aeschylus depicted in the *Oresteia* as necessary for the appropriation of an individual self capable of functioning in a city-state. The *Homeric Hymn to Demeter*, which reflects the Mysteries, evokes a sense of primal union and fusion with a ritual, matricentric world, suggesting that this union is not something from which one needs to defiantly escape to assert oneself, but acts rather as an empathic continuum through which differentiation can occur.

The Hymn probably was composed orally a few decades after Homer's *Iliad* and *Odyssey* and continued in oral and written composition until just before the 5th century. It is therefore a product of a patriarchal polis as well as of an earlier period that embraced a more permeable consciousness. The Hymn and the ancient Greek Eleusinian Mysteries that form the ritual context for it celebrate and worship the grief, rage, and ecstasy of the grain mother Demeter as she loses and regains her daughter, the *kore*, to *Aidoneus* (Hades), God of the underworld. This myth and the ritual supporting the Mysteries were so powerful in Greece that for hundreds of years people came to Athens yearly to march to Eleusis in order to participate in an initiation that they believed would grant them eternal life in the Isles of the Blessed. The immortality promised was deeply joined to Demeter's love for her daughter, as if the very energy that set in motion the seasonal cycles emanated from the emotional intensity of the mother-daughter bond. Surprisingly, it was precisely through the eternal recurrence of the seasons as embodied in the figure of Demeter and Persephone that initiates felt the possibility of not only collective but individual immortality.

Carl Jung's insight into how archetypes function to promote individuation was in fact founded in the mother-daughter relationship as seen through the Hymn and the Mysteries. He says:

> A woman lives earlier as a mother, later as a daughter. The conscious experience of these ties produces the feeling that her life is spread out over generations – the first steps towards the immediate experience and conviction of being outside time, which brings with it a feeling of immortality. The individual's life is elevated into a type, indeed it becomes the archetype of woman's fate in general … An experience of this kind gives the individual a place and meaning in the life of the generations, so that all unnecessary obstacles are cleared out of the way of the life-stream that is to flow through her. At the same time the individual is rescued from her isolation and restored to wholeness. All ritual preoccupation with archetypes ultimately has this aim and this result.
>
> (Quoted in Kerenyi, 1967, p. xxxi)

What Jung suggests is that in the awareness of the lifestream flowing through us, we lose our sense of isolation and feel the wholeness of the self, which is always connected, for him, with the collective psyche. What initiates may have felt was that *Kore*'s separation from and rejoining Demeter as a queen equal to her mother, yet holding her own domain, provided them with the possibility of having a sense of their own agency, power, and immortality precisely through celebrating the ritual of seasonal cycles. The very anthropomorphizing of the seasons into divine female figures who were never fully at home in Olympianism but maintained their status as older nature figures as well, may have allowed a possibility for a belief in a personal agency that could simultaneously maintain its sense of intimate connection with the cosmos.

The language of the Hymn operates at two levels, the first of which works through image and metaphor, implicitly evoking a matristic world of cyclical, agricultural ritual. The second works on the linear narrative level and tells a story of patriarchal domination involving the rape of the *kore* (Persephone) by Aidoneus (a name for Hades) and the attempt of Zeus and Helios to coax and coerce Demeter into accepting the loss of her daughter forever. Demeter refuses, and in her power as a nature goddess she creates a famine on the land, which compels Zeus to grant her her wish of having her daughter back with her for at least part of the year.

The rape of Persephone by Aidoneus expresses what may well be a predominantly patriarchal perception that to separate from the mother and the cyclical world she represents requires an act of violence, and that death is horrifying because it is the equivalent of self-dissolution back into that matricentric world. But the matristic, symbolic level of the text shimmers through this patriarchal overlay of rape and disjunction. The images connect and interweave, joining not only female divinities, but merging those divinities with natural elements in a nonhierarchical way. This metaphorical connection moves into the empathic flow of feeling and identification among Demeter, Persephone, Hecate, and other female presences in the poem, all in the context of seasonal cycles of birth and decay.

The opening of the Hymn suggests an acquiescence on the part of the powers of nature to the descent of the *kore* as part of a magical and fertile cycle of transformation. What appear to be oppositional or unrelated notions actually coalesce through images that move within a relational field, flowing together even as they come into focus as distinct. Each image of life at the beginning of the Hymn is also an image of death. The golden wheat Demeter holds is synonymous in Greek with the sickle that harvests it (*chrusaoros*). The narcissus in its hundred-headedness gleams wet with fertility, yet Hades, who mirrors the narcissus' multiplicity through his name here, *Polydeuktes,* "receiver of many," is the god of death in the underworld. This narcissus, the seducer of the *kore*, which will lead to her death and fertilization through her own plucking of it, is honored in its holiness by all mortals and immortals. Even the sea, the earth, and sky smile in the sweetness of its scent. Smiling, an opening of the mouth into a breaking of order, preludes the gaping of the earth that will allow the *kore*'s disappearance. The word for gape in Greek is *chazdo*, reminding us of the *xaos*, or chaos, from the same linguistic root.

The *kore*'s name is associated with the buds of wheat plants (*korai*). Her face is described as a bud about to bloom, and her playmates are described as blossoms. As she reaches out with both hands *thambas* ("amazed," a word which also implies "being struck with ecstasy") to take the *athurma* (translated "toy," but also having connotations of an object of magical transformation), we sense that she is caught up in a transformative event of death and rebirth, and that speaking ritually and metaphorically, she draws to herself her own destiny. Persephone is the blossom. The *leimon* or "meadow" is a space of pleasure, but also of death in Greek myth. It also means "female genitalia." To read through the images then, as the "bloom" of the narcissus is plucked from the meadow, the virgin is deflowered and the genitalia opened to disclose the yawning chasm which is the original place of birth and death, the womb of mother earth from which we all come and into which we all return.

Although the narcissus can be interpreted as evoking the phallic and aggressive nature of Polydeuktes, "the receiver of many," it is not simply phallic in the male, aggressive, raping way that one might assume. Although one might say that the hundred-headedness of the flower expresses an overdetermined phallic exuberance, it is equally possible that its multiple, receptive nature has female connotations. Further, flowers in Greek myth when they are associated with males have connotations distinctively other than phallic aggression. Hyakinthos and Narcissus himself in fact were originally beautiful young men who were turned into flowers at their tragic deaths – Hyakinthos, because Apollo, who loved him, killed him in error; Narcissus because he drowned trying to embrace himself in love. Both these myths appear to be similar in their themes of vulnerable, youthful beloveds who die though the medium of a mirroring, identifying love.

The *kore*, in reaching for the narcissus in desire to pluck it from the earth, will also in this potential act pluck herself from her childhood and her connections with her mother and grandmother in their guise as earth mothers. She is able to do this through longing for a beauty that mirrors her own, thus gaining strength through this longing to move into a new and sexual stage of life that is identified with mortality. As with Narcissus, her own "narcissism" (which for a contemporary self-psychologist would be considered healthy and psychologically necessary in her pubescent journey) indirectly brings about her death, and there is a question as to whether she will ever rise again.

However, since she is both taken into her grandmother Gaia and is called up again through the will of her mother Demeter, her death has different implications from those of Narcissus or Hyacinthus. For she rises again as all flowers, all fertility in the seasonal cycle. In this sense her death is a death of power, not of loss, which allows the seasons to keep turning through the mediation of earth goddesses.

How, then, does the narrative level of the text, which is so violent, makes sense? Aidoneus comes up in his golden chariot with his immortal horses and seizes the *kore* away as she "screams laments," *iachese orthia*, "unwilling." Surely this is a rape. But once again, we are working on both an implicit and explicit level. Implicitly, through the imagery, we feel irremediable, sudden, and violent separation. The earth opens, and shrill lamenting splits the sense of wholeness and serenity of a formally unified cosmos. This is the first time sound emerges in the poem and it is of a particular sort: *Iaxe* is the same word that is used of the cry of the Bacchantes as they go forward into the rite, or the tearing apart of live animals in the celebration of the fragmentation and eating of life that the world may renew itself. *Orthia* are shrill cries often connected with death laments. In other words what was whole has suddenly split with sound and gaping, and it has happened through a "snare," *dolos*, a deceit of mother earth herself. The maiden herself cries like a bacchant. And the sea, earth, and sky, all pre-Olympian animistic powers, have brought about the gaping through their own smiling acquiescence. The gaping is at once the mouth opening in the smile and the earth opening to receive the seed.

At this implicit level the images defy separation; they cannot be pulled apart. Flowers pluck flowers, and the generations are convoluted, springing and rounding back one on the other. The *kore* is in fact indistinguishable from her mother or her grandmother. According to other variants of the myth, it is impossible to tell whose mother is whose, or who gets raped. Demeter and Rhea have both been called the mother of the *kore*, Demeter is both a mother and daughter, and both Demeter and the *kore* have been thought to bear the same child (cf. Kerenyi, 1960/1967, pp. 132–133). It seems as if in this particularity of violence, time is struggling to be born, and the only way it can is through the recognition of violent separation, splitting apart of the whole into the halves of mother and daughter, or the older and younger parts of the female. In this way, the grieving of Demeter is understandable, not so much as the grieving of a mother for her daughter in today's individuated terms, but as a woman who has lost a younger part of herself as the generations come to be.

It is here that we conceive the violence of the diremption into death as a patriarchal overlay. For women, death, although it may be violent, is also closely joined with a sense of their own bearing cycles, and consequently, the seasons. On the symbolic, matristic level of the Hymn, death emerges as an organic process. The sense of the female individual self is an outgrowth of this grounding in eternal time. The brittleness of self felt in the violence of the patriarchal overlay may well reflect fear of dissolution into a nature that has no individuality. It is equivalent to the death of the ego – the self as agent. It is female acceptance of this through connection with the generations, as Jung says, that allows the distinction to occur without the rigidity of isolation. Women live and individuate within the context of an inevitable death that lies within, in their own cycles of birthing and weaning. Possible confirmation for this way of thinking about male and female attitudes toward death and the self is that in the Eleusinian mysteries a sense of immortality was so deeply fused with women that men who participated in their rituals "entered the figure of Demeter and became one with the Goddess" (Jung and Kerenyi, 1963, p. 140). Indeed, historical evidence indicates that even the male initiate regarded himself as a goddess rather than a god.

Sensing the metaphorical level of the text in the context of many of the mythic and linguistic associations available to the oral poet's collective awareness, one can see how Demeter, Kore, and Gaia are intricately webbed through images that embody cycles of death and renewal. Their intermingling and identification through myth and ritual, together with the webbed symbols of plants, divinities, and humans, bring us into a nonhierarchical world where distinctions emerge as meaningful only within the context of relational symbolic fields.

The mother-daughter relation itself moves into a permeable and vulnerable exchange of intimacy, in which Demeter can fully grieve her daughter's loss and equally rejoice together with her on her return after their prolonged dearth-full absence:

> hos tote men propanē mar omophrona thumon
> exousai
> polla mal allelōn kradien kai thumon iainon
> amphagapadzomenai. Acheon d'apepaueto thumos.
> Gethosunas, d'edechonto par allelōn edidon te.
>
> (The Homeric Hymn to Demeter, 1920, trans. H.G. Evelyn-White, [*Hom. Hymn. Dem.* 434–437])

> So did they then, holding the same-minded heart, melt each
> other's heart and spirit, both embracing and throwing their arms around each other many
> times. Their heart ceased from pain, and they received and gave to one another joyousness.
>
> (my translation)

The Greek here is almost impossible to render into English. *Amphagapadzomenai*, "Both embracing together and throwing their arms around each other," is a single word. *Allelōn*, "one another," is a single word. Their hearts seem now one, now two. The very word I translate as heart, *thumos*, expresses a kind of dynamic libidinous energy. There is the sense of their mingling and merging as one in their joy, not as two separate women only, but as parts of one.

Catherine Keller refers to this relational state as an empathic continuum. She states that "daughters then" (like Persephone) may learn to "differentiate themselves in and through an intimate bond with the universe" (1986, p. 151). Strangely enough, what this does is to allow the concept of a single, great Mother Goddess to become un-reified. No longer is she "an illusory projection of external omnipotence, upon which creatures unilaterally depend (the patriarchal ideal), but [as] a life force, indeed [as] a libido, internal to everything" (p. 151). The relation between Demeter, Persephone, Gaia, and the natural world is as Dionysian as the cries Demeter utters on Persephone's return – filled with sacrifice, filled with recurrence and yet filled with distinction in the continuum of the life cycle. The matristic level of the Hymn honors the recurring nonviolent yet grief-striking celebration of mortality in the eternity of continuance.

Feminist social psychologists Nancy Chodorow (1978), Carol Gilligan (1982), and others have studied the relationship between mother and daughter in today's familial contexts to formulate hypotheses about the way women conceive relationships and ethics differently from men. Jean Baker Miller and her colleagues at the Stone Center in Wellesley, Massachusetts, create theoretical and linguistic frameworks for the notion of relational being as they, in process together, understand it (Jordan, Surrey and Kaplan, 1991). Miller follows theorists who conceive the notion of the self as emerging out of an interpersonal field. Archaeologist Marija Gimbutas (1989), Riane Eisler (1987), and Lucy Goodison (1989) evoke relational being as they research pre-Mycenean societies to find evidence for the imminence in multiplicity of a "female sacred" in distinction to a single, transcendent Great Goddess, and for evidence of partnership governance rather than the political hierarchical model assumed by patriarchal thinking.

Relational being as it is put forth in the Hymn provides a powerful alternative to the self-in-crisis that the tragedians picture as being the necessary outcome of the repudiation of a matricentric world in the interest of developing will and agency. The term "being in relation" used by the feminist psychologists above demands as well that we give up concepts of self-formulation that suggest we move from merger with the mother to an ego autonomy that implies a reification of self if we are to feel safe enough to relate to others. Self in these constructs is usually correlated with ego. The anxiety of relating, in this model, apparently has to do with how much one can connect or empathize without losing a sense of self. The danger lies in the perception of relation as power-driven, where the "other" is likely to bind, limit, or control us. The fear of losing ourselves in relationship, according to this view, arises from an imagined pre-oedipal stage with our mothers in which fusion with her implies a stated dependency and weakness, making us likely to lose any sense of ourselves as distinct. Like the ancient Greek tragedies we have discussed, there is nothing in the above view, which is dedicated to ego separation, to suggest the possibility of remaining in a transitional space that might allow us to become distinct without becoming simultaneously separate.

For Miller and others mentioned above, it is unlikely that a core self can be developed outside the relational field. Our sense of knowing occurs in an emotional field, in a "between" in which both persons are participants. Mutual empathy replaces the term self. The goal of development, which takes as its model the mother-daughter relationship, is the development of mutually empathic relationships. This development replaces the goal of self-development. That does not mean that self does not develop, but it only becomes present in the context of mutuality, as one is "*present and moving* with the other(s) in creating a relationship dynamic and shaping a relational context" (Surrey, Kaplan, and Jordan, 1990, p. 2) No longer, then, are we to think in a paradigm of separation and individuation of self in a static field, but rather of relationship and differentiation in process, in a space-time continuum. This is in accord with many other disciplinary movements, most especially mirroring some of the new developments in physics:

> Connection has replaced self as the core element or the locus of creative energy of development. This approach reverberates with the new physics of subatomic particles which exist only in relation ... (they are) involved but do not contain each other.
>
> (p. 3)

These feminist theories of relational being complement the work of intersubjectivists, Jungians, and archetypal psychologists. The *Homeric Hymn to Demeter* supports and opens all their respective languages by speaking in images that can help us to feel our own extended embodiment in the post-Cartesian world. However, what the Demeter/Kore story brings us that neither intersubjectivists, archetypal psychologists, object-relations psychologists, nor feminist social psychologists have, and which Jung only implies, is the primary physicality through which we experience this sense of relation.

Insofar as women are creatures with orifices out of which we bleed, through which we admit seed, and from which we bear our own flesh and blood, we live at a level of fusion, symbiosis, and osmosis. That is, we live in the body knowledge that we are permeable. It is not just that we care for and relate, it is that we sense ourselves as being mixed with the next and previous generations. We feel the blood transfusing, or pouring through, into, and across generations. When we relate, there is a sense of physicality being exchanged, as we nourish each other and are nourished, we sense it at the level of feeding, of symbiosis (cf. Lowinski, 1992).

This sense of pouring through, into and out of, like the rhythmic waves of the sea, both senses distinctions and erases boundaries. As waves move across the sand, each time erasing the marks they left before, as billows and white caps meet and cross each other in surging and ebbing, as the undertow pulls back to thrust forward again, so are women aware of differences in qualities and rhythms, of myriad distinctions in our substance, washing, erasing, and once again creating endlessly and cyclically. We can move with endless, minute differences because we know in our deepest body nature that our substance is the same.

The *Homeric Hymn to Demeter* dreams us further into a way of being in relation, both with ourselves and those around us, deepening our sense of self in relation to a collective soul-making with others, past, present, and future. Insofar as being in relation always engages us in process, we feel the flow of immortality running through our veins.

The text of the Hymn brings this awareness to us in the way we engage in its symbols. We do so, feeling them as transitional objects, as what keeps us webbed in interdependence. The maternal container Gaia, through which all things live and breathe, and in which they find distinction, is developed through the Hymn into an "aesthetic experience" as Bollas (1987) defines it (p. 31). To dwell on the Demeter-Persephone relation in the Hymn is to feel fully how mother-infant relating is, in Bollas' words, "the first human aesthetic" (p. 31). Moving through the creative play of transitional space, as Winnicott defines it, such an aesthetic can crystallize "time into a space where subject and object appeared to achieve an intimate rendezvous" (p. 31). Just as the transitional object, as Winnicott says, allows the safe connection to be made between inside and outside worlds for the infant and opens the space of play that moves us into an expanded symbolic, aesthetic space as adults, so do the symbols here place us in connection with the text in a deeply felt and related way that lets us feel our very existence and sacred presence in the world. They also allow us at once to connect and to differentiate from the world. The goal is not to move into separation and autonomy, nor to leave the symbol behind, but to stay with such transitional objects, allowing them to grow more complex and interwoven. "A widening play of image and relationship will create both a more spacious world and a bigger self, never lacking the 'transitional objects' that liberate us from dependency" (Keller, 1986, p. 154).

Staying with the symbol as it transforms means relating to it in an organic and embodied sense. It means that the symbol as it becomes unique and specific to us is also becoming flesh, becoming a part of ourselves. This attention to the tending of symbols has profound healing potential in the therapy room. "Images are here to get 'embodied and ensouled, not literalized and idolized'" (Keller, 1986, p. 251).

Keller suggests that staying with the world of symbols in such a way that they continue to form the strong threads that hold us to the world and as well as to ourselves may be by becoming as a child:

> The child's intimation of immediate connection with the world does not return her to the womb. Oceanic feeling can permeate and moisten without drowning … how can we reclaim without regression the fluid boundaries of the child? Perhaps the first step or plunge, happens by letting ourselves feel how we are already there; by trusting that we already are distinctive in and through our connections; that we are already being empowered in our very permeability; that something in us is never cut off, never lost. We can feel the oceanic feeling surging through us, this moment ebbing and flowing, not threatening.
>
> (Keller, 1986, p. 147)

In sum, the Greek patriarchs appeared to need to radically separate in order to feel autonomous and in so doing prepared the way for later psychological theories of autonomy. The *Homeric Hymn to Demeter*, however, through its poetic embodiment of a self-in-relation, female permeability, and the complex interweaving of its images enhances the languages of feminists, and intersubjectivists, who are willing to consider transitional space as one that opens the possibility of attaining self-coherence through increasing interdependency. The visualization of the space of the Hymn itself provides an imaginal way of conceiving the therapy room as a maternal container that seeks through the imagery of the patient to develop this interdependent and multiply coherent self.

References

Alford, C.F. (1992). *The Psychoanalytic Theory of Greek Tragedy*. New Haven, CT: Yale University Press.

Bollas, C. (1987). *The Shadow of the Object: Psychoanalysis of the Unthought Known*. New York: Columbia University Press.

Chodorow, N. (1978). *The Reproduction of Mothering*. Berkeley: University of California Press.

Devereux, G. (1985). *The Character of the Euripidean Hippolytos: An Ethno-psychoanalytical Study*. Chico, CA: Scholar Press.

Dodds, E.R. (1951). *The Greeks and the Irrational*. Berkeley: University of California Press.

Downing, C. (ed.) (1994). *The Long Journey Home: Revisioning the Myth of Demeter* and *Persephone for Our Time*. Boston, MA: Shambhala.

Eisler, R. (1987). *The Chalice and the Blade: Our History, Our Future*. San Francisco, CA: Harper.

Euripides. *Bacchae* (1974) (E.R. Dodds, ed.) London: Oxford at the Clarendon Press.

Foley, H.P. (ed.) (1994). *The Homeric Hymn to Demeter: Translation, Commentary, and Interpretive Essays*. Princeton, NJ: Princeton University Press.

Gilligan, C. (1982). *In a Different Voice: Psychological Theory and Women's Development*. Cambridge, MA: Harvard University Press.

Gimbutas, M. (1989). *The Language of* the Goddess. San Francisco: Harper and Row.

Goodison, L. (1989). *Death, Women, and the Sun*. BICS Supplement #530. London.

Gouldner, A. (1965). *Enter Plato*. New York: Basic Books.

Hymn to Demeter (1920). *Hesiod, The Homeric Hymns and Homerica* (H.G. Evelyn-White, trans.) Cambridge, MA: Harvard University Press.

Jordan, J.V., Surrey, J.L., and Kaplan, A.G. (1991). Women and empathy: Implications for psychological development and psychotherapy. In *Women's Growth in Connection*. New York: Guilford Press, pp. 27–50.

Jung, C.G. and Kerenyi, C. (1963). *Essays on a Science of Mythology: The Myth of the Divine Child and the Mysteries of Eleusis* (1973). Princeton, NJ: Princeton University Press.

Keller, C. (1986). *From a Broken Web: Separatism, Sexism, and Self*. Boston: Beacon Press.

Kerenyi, C. (1967). *Eleusis: Archetypal Image of Mother and Daughter* (Ralph Manheim, trans.) Princeton, NJ: Princeton University Press. (Original work published in 1960.)

Lowinski, N.R. (1992). Stories *from the Motherline: Reclaiming the Mother-daughter Bond, Finding Our Feminine Souls*. Los Angeles: Jeremy P. Tarcher.

Riker, J.H. (1997). *Ethics and the Discovery of the Unconscious*. Albany, NY: State University of New York Press.

Segal,. C. (1981). *Tragedy and Civilization: An Interpretation of Sophocles*. Cambridge, MA: Harvard University Press.

Segal, C. (1982). *Dionysiac Poetics and Euripides' Bacchae*. Princeton, NJ: Princeton University Press.

Segal, C. (1986). *Interpreting Greek Tragedy: Myth, Poetry, Text*. Ithaca, NY: Cornell University Press.

Simon, B. (1978). *Mind and Madness in Ancient Greece*. Ithaca, NY: Cornell University Press

Slater, P.E. (1968). *The Glory of Hera: Greek Mythology and the Greek Family*. Boston, MA: Beacon Press.

Sophocles (1973). *Sophocles I: Oedipus* the *King* (D. Grene, trans.) *Oedipus at Colonus* (R. Fitzgerald, trans.), *Antigone* (E. Wyckoff, trans.) Chicago: University of Chicago.

Sophoclis Fabulae (1975). (A.C. Pearson, ed.), *Ely House*, London: Oxford University Press.

Stolorow, R.D., Brandchaft, B., and Atwood, G.E. (1987). *Psychoanalytic Treatment: An Intersubjective Approach*. Hillsdale, NJ: Analytic Press.

Stolorow, R.D., Atwood, G.E., and Brandchaft, B. (eds.) (1994). *The Intersubjective Perspective*. Northvale, NJ: Jason Aronson.

Sullivan, H.S. (1940). *Conceptions of Modern Psychiatry*. New York: Norton.

Surrey, J.L., Kaplan, A.G., and Jordan, J.V. (1990). *Empathy Revisited*. (Work In Progress #40.) Wellesley, MA: The Stone Center, Wellesley College.

Thucydides (1951). *The Peloponnesian War* (J.H. Finley, Jr., ed.). New York: Modem Library.

Part III

Case Studies: Myth and Psychoanalysis

Chapter 10

Imaginal Psyche in Psychotherapy

10.1 Mary

I once taught a class entitled "Women, Myth, Culture" at the Newberry Library in Chicago, one of the five remaining private humanities research institutions in the country. The course was open to students from other colleges in addition to my own. One of those students, whom I had not met previously, asked to come to my apartment the first day of class and talk to me. I was surprised at her boldness, and I granted her request.

She entered without the usual niceties of small talk, sat down immediately, and told me the story of her life. She started by saying that she had been gang raped by her four brothers when she was nine or ten, and that one day, when her mother took the family on vacation leaving her alcoholic husband at home, he set fire to the house and burned himself up in it.

I was not a clinician at that time and had no idea how to respond to this alarming confession. Mary's was not a story likely to be told by students to professors at any time, let alone at first meeting. Fearing my own inadequacy of response, I reflected to her my sense of what a terrifying story this was and how she must have suffered. She replied without emotion, "Oh I don't remember any of it. Others told me." I said, in astonishment, "You don't remember any of it??" She said again with almost no visible expression, "No. I only remember the things that happened before I was born."

I had the shivery sense one gets on hearing a ghost story. What could she mean by saying she remembered only what had happened before she was born? Was she living out of some deep

DOI: 10.4324/9781003340751-13

web of meaning that was helping to keep her alive? I entertained the thought that something beyond ordinary time and immediate human understanding must be holding her. The story of Hermes comes to mind, of his creating the lyre and then singing about his own parents' conception of him as if he were there at the time.

I was too startled to ask Mary anything more. I was aware that she wanted to stay close to me and I was deeply drawn to her. Why was I so deeply affected? One stormy night, as we were walking back up to the library from downtown watching the heavy snowflakes catching the light from the old-fashioned street lamps as they swirled about us, she stopped suddenly in front of a small shop where the highly glazed black pots of Maria Martinez, a well-known Native American artist were displayed. Mary seemed mesmerized, staring at a sign in the window, and said in an awed voice, "Those pots were made by MARY!" Since she did not know of the potter at all, I was struck by the intensity of her exclamation. I wondered if perhaps she thought that she herself had made the pots. I had the eerie sense that she had been swept up into another world, where she was a part of all the "Marys" in the world. She seemed in a trance.

When final research papers were due at the end of the course, Mary handed in a lengthy comparative paper on mother goddesses in different cultures. It was outstanding, except that it was missing references. When I asked her if, perhaps, she had forgotten to hand them in, she stared blankly at me and said: "I didn't use any."

I could have taken this as a bold-faced lie but, again, I couldn't shake the strange feeling that she lived in another world where her mind had full access to this material. Mary awakened me to the idea that there could be other fields of consciousness that most people can't perceive, but that seem to have a sense of viridity about them. They go beyond the ordinary into the extraordinary and seemed to sustain Mary and to give her a home. Her access to them appears to have arisen from un-survivable trauma and to have kept her alive and even sane enough to function both in and yet beyond a more mundane reality. The energy of Mary's force field had swept me in as well. We were held in a kind of vortex.

But was her present world a result of her terrible trauma, and therefore delusional? Or could she be dwelling in a space of "extraordinary knowing" (Mayer, 2007) that has its own authenticity and meaning that we are not usually privy to? (cf. Eshel, 2006, Kalsched 2013) Perhaps she lived rooted in the comfort of C.G. Jung's collective unconscious, in a world of archetypes that having a sense of the infinite and eternal, gave her some solace, as they did for Jung himself (1965a). This kind of reality is further amplified in Jung's conversations with Wolfgang Pauli who relates quantum physics with analytic psychology suggesting that there are worlds that are far beyond our comprehension (Jung and Pauli, 2014). I explored Bohm's world of implicate order, and Sheldrake's notion of morphic resonance, and returned to Freud himself to find that he also was quite aware of the paranormal and the uncanny unknown. Wherever Mary lived, and whatever experiences she called up such that she didn't "use any references," and whether or not she was lying, I was enthralled. I felt as if I myself recognized and was familiar with her world. For me, it existed as a shadow land, imbuing me with a deep longing for ultimate answers.

I do not know what happened to Mary and I never heard from her again. But it is in large part because of her that I was driven to study depth psychology and psychoanalysis in search of answers to the mysteries of the human psyche.

Mary's story stands as a prelude to what I learned in my early psychotherapy practice from two remarkable patients, who seemed to inhabit fields of a strange and intense energy like hers. In my experiences with them as a clinician, I had the chance to immerse myself intersubjectively and to discover more about how and why remaining with them in such fields could bring about healing for each of us (cf. Kohut, 1991, p. 545).

10.2 Liza

Liza came to see me in a state of traumatic shock, having witnessed a bad car accident. In the accident, a car coming in the other direction on a steep mountain road had skated on ice right next to her own car and slipped off the cliff into the crevasse below. A mother and her two small children were in the car. The mother and her son had been killed; the three-year-old daughter lived but was in serious condition at the hospital.

Liza knew she must be in shock, but she could not experience her own trauma. She told me first she had done a visualization exercise in a group about a month prior to the accident where she was asked to imagine someone bringing her a gift. The gift was brought to her by an old wise man, who handed her a rose. The name of the woman killed in the accident was “Rose.” It was this synchronistic connection, as Liza explained it, that made her know she had to come into therapy. She said to me, “A woman, Rose, died for me. That is the meaning. Her death was my gift.”

Liza’s connection seemed odd to me, although I felt it gave her some sense of meaning regarding the tragic, meaningless event she had witnessed. I waited. She began to relate her dreams. One told of a child, a female child, who was drowning. Liza kept attempting to save her and, being unable to, she would wake in terror. Sometimes it was one of her two sons that was drowning. That was worse. She also dreamed of driving up a cliff road and then down the hill into deep water – of calling for help and having no one see it was an emergency.

Liza was the daughter of a clinically depressed mother who had attempted suicide at least twice during the period when Liza was growing up. Her father was successful, but compulsive and perfectionistic, perhaps in an effort not to “crack up” over any of his own dismal past with violent and alcoholic parents. He put all his desires for perfection into Liza. Liza was a pretty, but quite tight-shouldered woman, who appeared to wear her muscles as a case around her body. Her neck was so taut and tense that one could see her muscles, veins, and tendons when she spoke. She was always perfectly groomed. The trauma of the accident had made her own unhappiness surface, and her dreams told me that she felt the younger part of her was on the verge of drowning. Perhaps the fact that the three-year-old daughter in the accident had been saved gave her some hope that she could save herself and break from her rigid physical and emotional encasements.

For several months after the accident she had witnessed, she was highly sensitive and hyper-alert to any possible catastrophe, terrified that every plane she heard overhead might crash, desperately afraid that "little plants may be drowning." She had a dream in which she was back at the scene of the accident, seeing a bicycle skid off the road. Unable to get an operator to call 911, she cried out in the dream, "Does anyone know how desperate I am?"

Liza lived in and through synchronicities, which she experienced frequently. However, this did not seem to mitigate her frequent crying spells, feelings of anhedonia, and desire to sleep all the time. Despite the fact that she realized she had a strong chance of an inherited predisposition to depression, she had refused any medication, saying that she wanted "to give this child (herself) natural childbirth." I decided to trust in her dreams and experiences of synchronicity, sharing in her conviction that they had meaning.

Early on, she told me of a strange incident with her son. He was doing a crossword puzzle ("which he never does") and asked Liza for the name of a bone in the forearm. Later that day he played a game of soccer, in which there was another boy playing who was missing an arm. Her child was wondering how this armless boy could play soccer. Not many moments after, the armless boy fell on top of her child, who broke the same bone in his arm the name of which he had been asking about for the crossword puzzle. Surely this was not a coincidence, Liza thought. It was too strangely synchronous and too close in detail to be so.

The second incident occurred when Liza was beginning to feel that she had married a man who was unable to nourish her. She had been trying to mend this marriage in every way she knew. One morning she walked into the kitchen, and one of her pottery wedding gifts slipped from her hands and broke. While this was explicable in terms of Liza's own ambivalence about the marriage, what was not so explicable was her walking into their bedroom later that day, hearing a crash, and finding that their wedding picture, which had hung on the wall ever since their marriage many years earlier, had simply fallen off and broken. Liza talked about how good it felt "when all these things came together." "It tingles," she said, "like being in an electrical field."

Liza felt more coherent, it seemed, by believing she lived in the presence of an energy field that picked up her own vibrations – as if her skin extended beyond herself – as if being in this field gave her a sense of structure and stability. They also gave her what she felt were important messages through images that were capable of helping her toward positive transformation. It was as if she did not have any home within her, given the false self she had been compelled to wear as a rigid shell, and so she found her home outside herself in being one with this extraordinary world (cf. Bohm (1980), on implicate order, and Coburn (2013) on complexity theory). This experience gave her considerable comfort and a sense of excitement and intense pleasure. In this way, she reminded me of Mary.

We might as clinicians talk about this in terms of dissociation from traumatic events in her past, and de-realization, but I felt that the images themselves that she lived with and created provided an aesthetic field that might lead us to her eventual embodiment. That is, rather than work to get rid of them so that she could be more grounded, they in themselves might help her to build herself.

One day she spoke to me about her love of butterflies, and her noticing of them at specific and important moments in her day. She began to hear mentions of butterflies in songs on the radio and to consider those moments highly significant as if there was an energic connection between her outside sightings of butterflies and her inner feelings. Butterflies landed on her sandwiches and flew into her window, as if they came of their own accord to make her feel better, she said. As I helped Liza to understand why she might feel so tense and tight, given her family background, I also encouraged her to feel these experiences fully.

On a succeeding day she came in with a butterfly dream. She had awakened in the dream to see a butterfly that was dark purple and black. She described it as "exquisite" and "like a pansy." She then found in her dream a small, purple butterfly. It was very frail and wilted from moisture. She began to take it inside her house, so that it would recover, but a friend in the dream suggested that she leave it outside to recover. The question for Liza was that she was not sure whether the butterfly was or was not a flower. If it was a flower and wet from moisture, it might have been better to leave it outside. If it was a butterfly with wet wings, it might have been better to bring it in to dry out. Liza noticed the next time she saw me that there were black and purple pansies growing in the flower bed right outside my office.

My own associations to this dream were that the first butterfly looked like a Mourning Cloak as well as the pansies growing outside my office. This larger butterfly announced the theme of grieving in the therapy. The little wilted flower/butterfly was a meshed image that was liminal for her. She fully identified with the image as if she herself was both flower and butterfly (perhaps what she was and what she wanted to become). I read the image as if she did not know whether or not it was in her best interest to come into my office and to grieve, or to remain rooted where she was, right outside. But even as a "flower," she was close to my office rather than elsewhere. As the butterfly with which she identified so strongly, it seemed she might dry out by coming inside. This dream had a paradoxical quality of outside/inside, as well as a transitional quality of identification with a fused object that if teased apart might bring her into a less watery place. Perhaps she needed to grieve before she could transform and fly.

Staying with the image of the butterfly helped it to become alive for both of us in the room without analyzing any psychological process behind it. It was a creature become numinous and substantial through her connections with it. I felt that staying with these images without interpretation would help to bring Liza into being and might give her more of a sense of self.

In the next dream, two months later, she saw a butterfly that was a "sage" green color, spread wide and flat on her "home page." She awoke with the phrase in her mouth: "Anything is possible." Eight months later, she came in looking very happy and excited, announcing that she had dreamed of a yellow butterfly attached to a blue flower that blew into the house on a wind and landed on "my hair or hand. I can't grasp it, but at least it is in my house. There seems to be the possibility of an 'airy garden.' The house is topsy turvy, but it doesn't stress me out. It feels okay."

Here, there is a clear differentiation from the earlier fusion. The 'sage' (wise) green butterfly in her dream suggested a possibility for her own growth, especially as it was on her "home page." The next dream, eight months later, of the yellow butterfly attached to a blue flower also showed a distinguishable separation of butterfly and flower both in their color and their type. This butterfly then sailed into the house of its own accord, promising "an airy garden," which I surmised might be a place where she could breathe and live on her own. She was becoming freer and she seemed more relaxed. She was about to be able to see herself as a butterfly, separated both in image and color from her first doubtful and ambiguous image.

Liza worked gradually to ground these images within her. Events happening beyond her perceived boundaries, at least in my empathic recognition and celebration of them with her, gradually gave her the sense that she had some coherence and substance. That these events were in fact happening to her and were real to her gave her the faith to feel authentic in their presence. As they were gradually taken in, these liminal experiences appeared to lose their quality of floating in the stratosphere and to engage with her in such a way as to create an integrated sense of self. It was as if she became a stronger node in the web of her own image making. It was as if the centripetal became the centrifugal, and that she was weaving herself into being.

I came to trust in Liza's butterflies. We wondered and wandered together in her fields of imaginal butterflies. One day, I felt moved to tell her the myth of Amor and Psyche, about the tasks Psyche had to perform to become free and to free both herself and Amor from nonpersonal archetypal forces. I also told her that Psyche, or "soul," was often represented in Greek vase painting as a butterfly. She told me later that this story, even though it did not come from her, this myth "carried" her.

Lisa's butterflies became a signpost to me of how the therapy was proceeding. I encouraged her to make them her very own in some way. She decided to create a ritual for herself. One day she came to see me saying that she had purchased some cocoons that were going to hatch into butterflies, and that she had been caring for them. She was going to arrange a ritual in which they would fly away. On the day of the ritual, two of the butterflies had apparently not survived. The others had flown as Liza set them free, but Liza's response to her act was to grieve their going rather than to celebrate their freedom. She appeared quite forlorn as if she had lost a beloved transitional object too early.

After this, she became increasingly determined to be unguarded about the deeper issues in her life that caused her pain. She faced the fact that she had never thought she could get angry with her father, and that his very occasional anger at her had devastated her. She took up at that point an aggressive sport through which she could express her anger at him, and this, together with work in the therapy room gave her the chance to see that she did not need turn her anger against herself. This brought her to a place of assertiveness, giving her inner energy to express her budding agency.

At around this time, she also began to have childbirth dreams. At first there were dreams of still birth, but, in a final dream, she found herself seated on a couch in front of a large window with an ocean beyond. A tidal wave rose and struck the window such that all the glass splintered into tiny pieces. All the water had suddenly disappeared. A girl-child on the floor, who was one-and-a-half years old (the number of years we had spent in therapy) began playing with the pieces. At first Liza was afraid, but then she observed that the glass pieces were more like harmless chunks. She lifted the child carefully into her lap and felt safe and whole.

It was after this dream that Liza decided that she could leave me. As she was leaving, she remarked that she had once again ordered butterfly cocoons and that some had already hatched and flown. She rejoiced in their leaving and was able to grieve and rejoice in her own leaving of me. This was the dream in which she could let go of her trauma regarding the accident she had witnessed. Her trauma had fused her own terrified young child-self with the little three-year-old girl injured in the accident. And the "Rose" (the name of the dead mother in the accident) she had been given by the wise man, which she visualized as a gift for her to find herself, had been fully accepted.

I felt in my work with Liza that greeting and engaging in the liminal spaces she believed she lived in already made her feel held by me in an open space of play where she could experience her own assertiveness without feeling that I would breakdown or become depressed like her mother. I became a safe cradle, a cocoon, from which she could grow wings and fly freely into an increasingly satisfying and expanding circle of relationships.

Living with Liza in these symbolic spaces and believing her images to have substantial reality felt to me as if we were moving together in a liminal reality. Greeting what she thought of as synchronicities and holding her experiences with open arms transformed butterflies into real soul spirits who held part of Liza safe until she could form her own wings. In doing so she became embodied and could relax the armor that shielded her own sense of despair and emptiness. In this therapy I became a nourishing mother and was able to nourish her imaginal world until she was able to fully believe in it, knowing it had been shared. The sense of reality came from her own belief in her own aesthetic being, as if she had created herself as poem.

The sense of self that emerged from Liza's experience seemed multiply coherent, as if she had never fully broken connection with her original dream spaces, fantasies, and synchronistic experiences, but rather had developed stronger links through them to her own emerging sense of self. My sense was that Liza had become integrated precisely by maintaining and coming to trust the increasingly supple and strong connections to her imaginal environment.

I felt that with Liza I had to yield to an experience of living at the edges of places I experienced as disorganizing, inchoate, fantastic, and that frequently made me feel as if I were spinning in space. This is perhaps what Green means when he says that one as a therapist has sometimes to live "at the cutting edge of his own madness but that, in this way, he may enter into a creative and redeeming relationship with madness" (quoted in Eigen,

1981, p. 79). The therapist's owning of madness and ability to tolerate the patient's madness allows experiencing to "link with itself across periods of breakdown" (p. 80). This linking creates continuity without giving up the madness that alone can make us free. In doing this we allow the patient to engage in creative play within the transitional area of the therapy room. Tolerating and holding disruption and unintegration is in this way being a good-enough mother therapist to survive, thus birthing the patient through the act of not being destroyed oneself.

I came to believe that synchronistic experiences are native to Liza and people like her. They appear to find their psychic homes not in linear time, nor even in their bodies, but in imaginal spaces pointing to a mysterious beyond. The language in which they express themselves and the stories they tell are in themselves signs to me that there are valid, perceptible metaphysical fields of which we can become acutely aware. C.G. Jung's description of the psychoid realm, Sufi understandings of subtle body, Catholic beliefs in saints and angels, and a multicultural belief in ghosts all try to describe this realm of being. It is a liminal realm that envisions figures not fully flesh, yet not pure ether. This space contains in-between, but substantial presences that are tangible and that inform us, in trenchant ways, of further reaches of consciousness. Transitional experiences (Winnicott), Reverie (Bion), the analytic third (Ogden), self/selfobject relationships (Kohut), emotional dwelling (Stolorow), complexity theory Coburn), and non-linear dynamic systems theory are all partial descriptors for these experiences. Aesthetic forms like narrative, poetry, and myth can help us both to soar and to feel safely enfolded by such experiences, especially if we as therapists can provide a maternal surround for ourselves and our patients as we invite such forces into the room. But ultimately, it seems we must go beyond them if we are to glean more understanding of what such force fields are, and why certain of our patients, and perhaps even ourselves, traumatized or not, feel so attuned to them.

Holding securely to the belief and historical understanding that peoples in traditional cultures in fact experience wholeness precisely through such connections gave me the courage to engage in a world that I otherwise might have found illusory and that I feared might throw both me and my patients into a world of fragmented emptiness. My grounding in archaic Greek literature and myth, and my own personal therapeutic experiences allowed me to do so. I gradually became convinced that my absolute faith in the fantasies of the patient provided not a defensive but a genuine thread to reality and allowed me the empathic stance that could call upon Liza's psyche to weave itself into authentic relational being.

But it was crucial also to hold the therapeutic field in a way that Liza could grow and flourish. I understood this as an "infant mother psychosomatic field" (Eigen, 1996, pp. 80–81). For me, this field needed to find its own breath not only in the language of psychoanalytic theory, evocative as it is, but in the fields and meadows of an imagined natural environment. It was here that I could sense that Liza's fantasies were not manic, idealized defenses against an inner emptiness, but rather their own imaginal worlds, filled with a quality of sunlight, space, and a sense of interconnectedness that needed strengthening rather than rupturing. The good-enough mother of the therapy room, in this view, becomes a full and supportive maternal environment.

10.3 Amanda

As crucial as it was to bring Liza into embodiment and a sense of self, Amanda was seeking a path to disembodiment and death. She announced herself on the phone as a 60-year-old who had been free from cancer for seven years. She said she had a strange symptom that she needed to figure out: "Whenever something good happens," she said, "I get ringing in my ears. The person who referred me to you told me I should tell you my two cancer dreams. When I told the dreams to her, she said, 'How fascinating!' as if I were some kind of oddity!" Amanda then said to me, "You sound delightful. When you see me, you probably won't want to work with me." And again, to my warm and positive response, she said, "If you don't want to work with me, please say so. Am I bothering you?" I assured her she was not and made an appointment with her. My sense over the phone was of a warm, eccentric, and outspoken woman with a nice sense of humor who suffered from very low self-esteem and who did not want to be considered sick or crazy.

When I came out of my office to greet Amanda, I was stunned by her beauty. She was tall, with a long, horsey face and striking features, a model's figure, and the whitest of white hair tied into a soft bun on her head. She had an immediate, warm smile and a golden glow which drew me to her.

In our first session, during which I could not have taken my eyes off her if I had tried, she spoke almost without stopping. She explained that the reason she came into therapy was that she was "unable to have an a-ha experience about my present difficulties." The first difficulty turned out to be some peculiar reaction to electrical transformers outside her house – she just "felt funny." The second was severe heart palpitations which prevented her from going places she wanted to, such as to visit a dear friend. The third difficulty was a terrible ringing in her left ear, followed by heat in her heart and then a feeling of weakness. This, she repeated, occurred "when anything really good is about to happen to me."

Recently, Amanda had gone on vacation with her husband and had an attack severe enough to warrant her asking to go to the doctor, who could find nothing wrong with her anywhere. She knew her cancer had happened for emotional reasons, and she knew there was an emotional reason for this as well. Suddenly, and with the look of an eager, desperate child, she leaned forward and said, with great intensity, "Can you help me?" As a therapist still in supervision, I had no idea what to say. I answered in a bumbling kind of way: "I don't know yet. I'm not sure."

She brushed my comment off rapidly and continued:

> My first a-ha experience happened in my one and only visit to a psychiatrist, in which I reported to him that in hanging out the diapers one day I remembered something that happened when I was three years old. This was when my parents pulled in a strange girl from the street to take care of me. She had to

> sleep in my bed, and every night she would kick me into the wall. She said she would kill me if I ever told.

The psychiatrist had, according to Amanda, told her that she had lived her life feeling she was about to be killed all the time. She said she got that one figured out and didn't need to go back. "That was your only visit?" I asked. She answered that she could always figure out and control her own body, both physical and mental processes.

She said she had refused all medical treatment for cancer even though she had been given only a month to live. She had never taken chemotherapy and had worked on her cancer through imaging and drugs she had gotten from an old anthroposophist from Germany.

At this point in that first hour, I began to feel dizzy. Images clustered in confusion around me. Was I still standing by the laundry line, seeing little Amanda in her bed being kicked into the wall by a strange street child, or was I watching the look on her former psychiatrist's face when she walked out "with everything solved"? She gave me no chance to speak. Her words poured out with great intensity. She plunged into her two cancer dreams:

> 1. I am in a car and my first cousin Will is driving. We are in a tunnel that is blue and he is driving on the left side of the road. All the cars are careening around us. On my right I see water rising up higher and higher. It looks as if it has garbage floating in it. I put my hand in and the first thing I pull out is bacon rind. Then there is something gold. It is a watch. It has water pouring from it.

Without stopping, she interprets for me: "My will-my masculine side (left guides right) is on the wrong side of the road. *Time* is running out for *cure.*"

> 2. I am with an old school friend, whose parents, in the front seat, are arguing: "You drive," "No, you drive," "No, you drive – his/her, his/her, his/her." Then they look directly at

> me, and my school friend says to them: "Just shut up and drive." They drive into a split rail fence.

Amanda again interprets with no room for comment: "His/her, his/her directly to me means 'hysterectomy.' A couple of days later I began to hemorrhage and told my husband that if I needed a hysterectomy they should give it to me. He was surprised since I want my body whole and I have refused chemotherapy."

I am struck by Amanda's intelligence and by her remarkable ability to read her dreams. I can see her need for self-control. I begin to feel as if I have entered into another world. Amanda seems a kind of soothsayer interpreting her own dream oracles. I begin to feel as if I am floating – the room tilts back and forth, and I am suspended in a viscous space. I find myself at a loss to know what to say again, but try to hold my ground:

> Amanda, you are so clever at figuring out your dreams!

She continues,

> I'm intuitive. When I was two or three, I was at my grandparents' house, whom I loved – my parents didn't have a happy marriage – and I insisted on seeing my mother. They said I would see her later in the afternoon. I insisted that it be now. My father came and he was furious with me for making such a fuss about seeing my mother. He took me home. The door was locked and when we got it open we saw Mother lying face down on the floor with the gas turned on in the stove. The nurse from across the street helped. From that time on I knew I had to take care of my parents.

Amanda told me she was an only child of an only child. She was married young to someone her mother approved of, but whom she did not love, and who was mentally very ill. She had no children (which she attributed to divine grace), and divorced him. She then married a man with whom she had two children, whom she divorced when her five-and-a-half-year-old son told her that his dad kept locked file cabinets of photographs of a murderer raping and killing women. After that, she took care of her children by herself until they were grown.

Her mother had had a magnificent voice, tried out at the Metropolitan Opera auditions, and was invited to come to New York, but was prohibited by her own mother. Amanda had had one year of college and got a fellowship in the arts. Her fiancé and parents came to an exhibition of hers, thought little of it, and wouldn't give her the 50 dollars she needed to validate her fellowship.

I asked if her mother ever sang in the house. "Yes," she said, "She was always complaining of her heavy-chestedness, and I told her later that was her gift. When she sang, it was so loud, it rang over the whole house." Amanda made a gesture with her hands in front of her heart area, as if pumping.

She asked again if I could help her. I told her I thought she was lonely and that she told a heroine's story. I said it sounded as if she had always had to take care of everyone, and that she had a way of never being done in. She said, "I am a circumventor," in this way perhaps once again circumventing me. When I told her the hour was up, feeling that I had been of no use at all, Amanda announced that she wanted a hug and was immediately intimate. She said she felt she had found a good friend to whom she could tell everything.

My presence during this first session was as an empathic, captive, and fascinated audience. She appeared to want no active responses. She needed to talk, and she was clearly performing for me. I found myself caught up in her golden glow.

But when she walked out, I felt again that I was swirling in an unaccustomed space. My own ears were ringing. I had a strange sense of unreality (even the hug had seemed unreal). I felt as if I were in a Dali painting. Things floated everywhere. Amanda was both highly attractive and somehow hideous to me as well. She was also fully energizing. I felt she would be a great gift to work with because she might teach me as well how to die, since it was clear she had always been in control of everything (I was not surprised that she brought her own tissue).

At the same time, she appeared disembodied. There was a strange split (the split rail fence) between her clever, verbal interpretations, and her attempt at an embodied life. Her images themselves were disembodied. The stories she told about herself appeared to be carefully constructed, and she treated her dreams as oracle centers that could give her answers. but she was emotionally disconnected from them. I wondered if she had made up the story about being a heroine in everything to avoid the terrible pain and rage about never having been recognized for who she was, or given what she wanted, and for her dreadful mistreatment, which she seemed unable to acknowledge. Did she project her heroine story as her only way of being real? That her ear ringing happened in the same location where she was not permitted to go to take the scholarship suggested to me that what was really ringing in her ears was her mother's voice, which also was never allowed to find its own fullness in a profession. The heat in Amanda's heart, which brought weakness, and her arm gestures as if pumping when she recalled to me her mother's shame over her "heavy-chestedness" seemed a physical enactment to me of her not being allowed to ever fulfill her own dreams, as her mother also was prohibited from doing: "Whenever something good is about to happen to me, I get ringing in my ears."

I sensed again how split Amanda was and how much she yearned for unity. This was corroborated when she told me how much it meant to her to have been taken to a "Unity" service when she was young. When she told me she was a writer of inspirational poetry, a fountain of tears quite suddenly poured down her face. Was it my task to help bring the hidden pain to the surface? Would that make her whole? Or was it really "too late for the cure?" Would she listen to anything I had to say or was it entirely too threatening for her to be helped or guided by another? Perhaps she just needed to be listened to, to pour out her soul to me.

My psychiatrist supervisor would be expecting a diagnosis. It was still early, but dissociation with histrionic and narcissistic features all seemed to fit the bill from what I had learned. When I described the session, he shot questions at me, and was intimidating in his comments: What have been her illnesses? Surgeries? Is she taking hormones? Did they take her ovaries? What's her history with traditional medicine? What are the loss issues around the hysterectomy? He told me she was very strange not to have accepted chemotherapy. Was this a well-circumscribed delusional system? Did she have magical ideas of herself and others? Were there signs of mental disintegration? Did she prefer to be lost in the ozone? When I said I had only seen her once, he was a little kinder. But he insisted I take a full medical history.

The next time, I sat down dutifully with my pen and paper. "Did you have anything you wanted to ask me?" she said sweetly. "Yes," I said, and proceeded, though I felt that what I was doing was already going south. Once again, what could have been simple responses poured out in fiery floods. She told me of her sensitivity to magnetic fields, about her clairvoyance – about getting sick and dizzy on the bus up to Minneapolis to see a psychiatrist to have an MRI, and having to get off, only to find when turning on the radio at home that on the very corner where the psychiatrist had his office a man had shot five people.

When I asked her how she felt about her own clairvoyance, she said she did not revel in it, she just let it come. She then changed the subject and said: "I just got the blood crystallization test back from Germany that I had been waiting for. Do you want to hear it?" "Yes," I answered. "They say I had cancer on my pancreas which has gone, but now there is activity in the abdominal area. I don't want to be specific because," she said. "When people hear this, they just get out the shovel and get ready to bury you."

Obediently following my supervisor's advice, I questioned her directly on whether she still wanted to continue with alternative medicine and was not willing to have chemotherapy. She said under no conditions would she have chemotherapy or radiation because she had seen what it had done to her father. Also, she said, she was having no pain.

"Can you handle this?" she said sharply as she rose to leave. "Yes," I said, reeling at her news and overcome with sadness, but with a boldness that surprised me. I also felt sheepish as I glanced down at the empty pad of paper on my lap.

I believe Amanda mentioned fires and the impossibilities of quenching them in that session because she knew that nothing now would really put out the fire of her cancer. She said she had been enduring for a long time and was tired. But then she had told me with a big grin about a stick figure she had drawn unconsciously on a piece of paper: "It means 'stick it out,'" she said. I felt I needed to know my role in helping her to have as rich and meaningful a time in those hours with me as she could. I needed to know either how to help her to heal, or to die.

In the next session, Amanda said she wanted to figure out some things to sort out why she created physical symptoms that kept her from doing things she really liked. She told me the cancer was all over her head, stomach, intestines, and liver. She talked about how innately talented she was in her life and about all the good things that had happened to her. At one point she broke down crying and caught herself quickly. I asked her why she felt she had to hold back her tears. The sobs then reached deep down within her, but she pulled herself up again. She said she had never been able to do what she wanted in life. Then she told me about how everything had come to her that she had ever wanted. She told me that I, like her husband, had been sent by God. She also told me laughingly, upon leaving the session, that she always hated to leave here because she was sure it would look to others as if I had been beating her (she cried so much). How split she was!

In the next session, she told me of a little boy whom she had babysat when she was 12 years old who hanged himself from the window frame with a belt because his parents had made him go back to school when he didn't want to. She then told me of two friends who had died on her birthday. When I asked her what that meant to her, she said abruptly, "Nothing. It was just a coincidence." Why was she telling me these things? Was she anticipating her own death?

She then told me a dream and a story that was scarcely distinguishable from a dream:

> I dreamed I had fallen down a hole, and had come up with great difficulty, scraping my hands and knees. I hauled myself out and found myself in a beautiful meadow. Five monks were coming toward me; each tended to one of my five senses.

> One cleaned my knees and hands, one fed me, and so forth. As they left, I cried out to them to come back, but they did not turn around. Finally, one did, and beat on his heart three times, pointing to a crystal palace in back of him.

Amanda said she had this dream three times around the time she was 30 (from the way she talked it could have been the night before), when her mother and father were dying, and she said she was sure it meant that there was more to life than the five senses. She said the third time she had had the dream there was a woman standing there. When she asked who she was, the woman said, "I am yourself." She cried at this. When she later said she did not fear death, I reminded her of the dream and said she seemed to feel there was a fullness of spirit beyond the five senses, but she grew cold, and said all she knew is that she would have to "pass through fire." Once again, I felt that whatever side of Amanda I chose to support, I was not to venture it. She needed a listener.

In the following (and last) three sessions, Amanda decided she wished to concentrate on three unresolved issues in the times ahead that she wanted to get clear. She told me her husband tried to suffocate her by caring for her cancer, not understanding that it was the unresolved issues which mattered. I asked if she felt she had the space and solitude to work through them here. She said she did, that she had felt better ever since she had come here, and that she was particularly grateful that I had asked to see her poetry (which I had), as this was the first time she had looked at it herself in a long time. Then she told me she had written a parable:

> A man came and gave me a beautiful baby. I handed it back to him. He told me I could keep it because he saw I had a baby carriage (a place to put it). When I said I could not because the carriage was full, he said, "What's it full of?" She lifted up a corner of the blanket and said, "Garbage."

Amanda felt that she was so full of garbage that there was no room for her, the beautiful child. Would we have time to clean out the garbage? Is that what she wanted? Or was the garbage the cancer itself – did she feel herself as rivers running with garbage?

In the seventh and last session, when Amanda walked in, my sense was that she had spent hours making herself look beautiful. Her white hair was up in a bun, her face was skillfully made up; she was wearing a little black vest with stars and red flowers on it, embroidered with gold thread, that made me fantasize that this was the cosmos, this darkness, and that she was the emanation of that cosmos coming through as stars, on the boundary between living and dying. I remembered the story she told me about knowing that when she died, she would be a guardian angel for small, dying children. She came in with an envelope which I assumed were poems she was going to read me. She said she felt well and that she had had a good week. For the first time, ten minutes before the hour ended, she looked at the clock and said, "Oh, our time is almost up."

I said, "We have ten minutes. Would you like to read me your poems? Or would you like me to read them?" She replied, "I can read them or you can read them and send them back to me." I replied, "Does that mean you're not coming back next week?" She said, yes, she needed a break, she did not want to "dig" anymore, she just wanted to live on the surface of life, enjoying each moment as it came. She said she had resolved all her issues and figured out her symptom. She said it meant that there was a noise, namely "communication," that something needed to be said that was then boiling inside her heart, and that she had been able to do that here. That's why she had come. It was very valuable, and it was enough. She read me a poem about a hawk flying free, which later I was to read in the exact same words in a poem she had written about her father's death, also from cancer.

She asked if I thought it was right that she take leave of me, and she looked once again like a pleading child. I was stunned (but not surprised) that she would bring this up so late in the hour and with no forewarning. Nevertheless, I felt deeply that she really wanted to be free and that going into her life, even into her rage and grief at this point in her life, was no longer her need or desire. I told her after a long silence in which I searched her eyes and face that I thought she knew a great deal about herself and that she would do what she felt best.

My heart cried out for her to stay and be strong enough to let me help her die, to let me see her as she had seen her father die, so "gross and ugly." But I felt she could not tolerate my seeing her ugliness, or trust that I cared for her whether she performed or not. I did not know how to say this in the two minutes I had left with another patient coming. She hugged me at the door, and I told her I was here if she needed help. She thanked me and left.

When Amanda had told me of the medical report, I had felt all my clinical psychological intent drain from me. I felt the senselessness of diagnosis. How could I be that kind of therapist to someone who was dying? Why did I need to take a medical history? Why should I question whether or not she was engaged in magical thinking, whether she had a grip on reality, whether she was or was not psychotic or should have chemotherapy? Didn't she have a right simply to tell me her story? In the spinning of the space around us, the breaking of all boundaries of ordinary reality, Amanda was already part ghost, embodied as a very present absence. Her stories changed constantly. Told, then gone, perhaps never to be told again, she flitted from one to another and they shimmered away. I had relished them, felt them, believed in them and seen her through them. I had also felt the abyss around which they were created, wondering if she had enough of a sense of herself to even realize that she was grieving. Her constancy was indeed one of fluidity.

But she had held out her arms to me. I had leaned forward and listened, rapt, feeling her desperate loneliness. I had reached out my hands to her, ready to take hers and accompany her to the threshold of death. And then I was left in the ache of a gesture unmet, cradling a beautiful child whom I felt would never be acknowledged by the woman who was leaving her behind to escape from a body "baby carriage" that was always full of "garbage."

What was I, as a therapist, to do with this orphan without a body, this unrealized self that wants to live to her fullest and was left unredeemed – the hawk-angel who flies through the fire into death? (Was she hawk or a phoenix?) I was left with the burden of unsaying.

10.4 Heidegger, Soul, and the Liminal

Living in these intermediate spaces with my two remarkable patients, it was clear to me that Liza needed to sense her embodiment, and Amanda had to accept disembodiment. But they both lived in liminal, symbolic spaces weaving together body and psyche into a third imaginal field to which I was both witness and participant.

It was at this time in my early life as a clinician that I began to think diagnosis was only a negation of the sheer poetry of being. If I were to try to interpret Amanda's tapestry of images and pick them apart for their meaning, they would unravel, and Amanda would lose the fabric of the color and richness that formed a home for her. If her own anticipated death provoked her mind to hallucinate and to create a daemonic space between earth and whatever lies beyond, I needed to respect that. At these moments of staying with dying there is no pathology, because there is nothing to be healed. My supervisor called it "psychosis" and "magical thinking." I called it "soul."

The word soul lends credence to a person's integrity and removes the sense of pathology connecting with "psychosis," and "magical thinking." It allows the possibility for further richness and connection in liminal realms, within which we can sense a certain faith and sacredness that gathers meaning. In my own grief at losing Amanda ("she who must be loved"), I was deeply drawn to a late, poetic essay of Heidegger's, entitled "Building, Dwelling, Thinking" (1971). Heidegger writes in a poetic and philosophical language that evokes my sense of liminal experience with Amanda better than I can. I was moved especially by his explanation of "symptom" as both a "bridge," and a "dwelling." This added to my own sense of psychotherapeutic process as a dwelling together. This sensed, third field of connection between analyst and patient, flowing between them and beyond consciousness expresses to me the truth of the intersubjective emotional relationship. It reveals what is beyond the reach of ordinary understanding. It is also primarily about care and tending. Heidegger's language enhanced my understanding:

> The old word "*bauen*" which says that man is insofar as he *dwells*, this word "*bauen*," however, *also* means at the same time to cherish and protect, to preserve and care for, specifically to till the soil, to cultivate the vine. Such building only takes care—it tends the growth that ripens into its fruit of its own accord.
>
> (Heidegger, 1971, p. 147)

At the moment that Amanda told me about her cancer spreading, I had put down my pencil from dutifully taking my medical record, and the space in the room grew different. The realm of duty, of what was appropriate, of what should be done, fell away. It was just us, there together, stripped and facing a reality so unknown and so palpable that there was no more acting, no more trying, no more being in that world where one fixes, molds, and tries to change. In that moment we were "dwelling" (Heidegger, 1971). In that moment, I was caring. And in that caring, there was a sense of freedom and of peace. And there was a bridging in which the space between us became thick, and in which the location of our bodies created a space for gathering: "To dwell, to be set at peace, means to remain at peace within the free, the preserve, the free sphere that safeguards each thing in its nature. *The fundamental character of dwelling is this sparing and preserving*" (Heidegger, 1971, p. 149). Perhaps in this way there was a saving and a very preserving of who Amanda was. "To save really means to set something free into its own 'presencing'" (Heidegger, 1971, p. 150). For Amanda, it was to be set free and like a hawk, to fly beyond.

Heidegger's words capture for me the quality of Amanda's journey out of her body and into death. In her spinning of dreams and visions, she catalyzed a vibrant energy that swept me up into her own particular imaginal sensibility, and in doing so I felt that she was gathering me into the truth of her very being. I was not only dwelling with her emotionally but she was enchanting me into a mysterious beyond where I felt just on the threshold of an answer to the riddle of life and death.

"Mortals dwell in that they initiate their own nature – their being capable of death as death – into the use and practice of this capacity so that there may be a good death" (1971, p. 151). We cannot dwell with the four-fold of earth, sky, divinities, and mortals by merely staying on earth, or under the sky: "Dwelling itself is always a staying with things" (Heidegger, 1971, p. 151). "The bridge is never first of all a mere bridge and then afterward a symbol" (p. 153). "The location is not already there before the bridge is … Rather a location comes into existence only by virtue of the bridge … only things that are locations in this manner allow for space" (p. 154).

Staying in this space with Amanda was in itself a symbolic gathering – like the bridge that gathers the banks on either side that emerge as banks only as the bridge connects them. The space between life and death felt like a space of disembodiment and derealization, where phantoms and ghosts disregarded the comfortably identifiable dwellings of dream, fantasy, and reality, sifting back and forth without boundaries. Her stories came in tangents with no regard for grammar, or the linearity of time, not saying whether they were story, or history, or where they came from or vanished to. The space was embodied, yet without a body. We danced together over an abyss, scattered, multiple, fragmented. Locations fell away and needed to be gathered anew in the space that she and I were among.

Beneath all of this was a constant weeping. Like a basso continuo, it was the one sound that was continuous and connected everything. But it was so much in the background that we scarcely heard it until the hours were up and she left with the visage like Agamemnon's, swollen, rough, and rutted with tear stains.

Understanding and living in the liminal had not in fact prepared me to watch a patient go fully into a space where she could leave her body behind. In her process of dying, there was no particular relation to the unconscious. It felt more like transcendence, a sense of a soul gathering itself to set itself free from her body.

This is a state the mystics describe as an alchemical stage in which the soul is rising to the divine through the *unio mystica – a mystical union.* "The psychological interpretation of this process leads into regions of inner psychic experience which defy our powers of scientific description" (Jung, 1966b Vol. 13, para. 482). More than that, like the word "self" itself, it defies any description at all.

References

Bohm, D. (1980). *Wholeness and the Implicate Order.* London: Routledge.

Coburn, W.J. (2013). *Psychoanalytic Complexity: Clinical Attitudes for Therapeutic Change* (Psychoanalytic Inquiry Book Series). London: Routledge.

Eigen, M. (1981). The area of faith in Winnicott, Lacan and Bion. *International Journal of Psychoanalysis* 62: 413–433.

Eshel, O. (2006). Where are you, my beloved? *International Journal of Psychoanalysis* 87(6): 1603–1627.

Heidegger, M. (1971). Building, dwelling, thinking. In Hofstadter (trans.), *Poetry, Language, Thought.* New York: Harper Colophon, pp. 145–162.

Jung, C.G. (1965). *Memories, Dreams, Reflections.* New York: Random House.

Jung, C.G. (1966a). The psychology of the transference. In R.F.C. Hull (trans.), The *Collected Works of C.G. Jung* (Vol. 16) (2nd ed.). Princeton: Princeton University Press. (Original work published in 1954.)

Jung, C.G. (1966b). The Philosophical Tree. In R.F.C. Hull (trans.), *The Collected Works of C.G. Jung* (Vol. 13). (2nd ed.). Princeton: Princeton University Press, para. 482, pp. 348–349. (Original work published in 1954.)

Jung, C.G. and Pauli, W. (2014). *Atom and Archetype: The Pauli/Jung Letters, 1932–1958* (C.A. Meier, ed.). Princeton: Princeton University Press.

Kalsched, D. (2013). *Trauma and the Soul: A Psycho-spiritual Approach to Human Development and its Interruption*. London: Routledge.
Kohut, H. (1991). Kohut and the search for the self. Vol. 4. In P. Ornstein (ed.). *Introspection, Empathy and the Semi-circle of Mental Health.* Madison, CT: International University Press, pp. 537–567.
Mayer, E.L. (2008). *Extraordinary Knowing: Science, Skepticism and the Inexplicable Powers of the Human Mind.* New York: Bantam Books.

Chapter 11

Psychoanalysis as Metamorphosis

11.1 Reclaiming the Mythic Depths of Human Experience

Throughout this book, I have invited you into a way of being that weaves together experiences of the conceptual and the imaginal to suggest the existence of a world that lies both beyond and within us and can help gather us together, both in our daily lives and in our therapeutic encounters.

From my own childhood life of fantasies as they meshed with bizarre, traumatic, and actual experiences during World War II, to my mother's death, which threw me into a melancholia that could only be "just" as Freud described, I was led beyond the personal to the archetypal world of Jung's collective unconscious, the mythic world of Neumann's comparative mythology, and the maternal aesthetic idiom of Christopher Bollas – a place where "The object is pursued to surrender to it as a medium that alters the self, where the subject-as-supplicant now feels himself to be the recipient of enviro-somatic caring, identified with the metamorphoses of the self" (Bollas, 1987, p. 14).

Bollas' transformational object world allowed me to feel justified in my strong feeling of immersion in a transcendent nature where I felt held and surrounded, as if at once in my mother's arms, and yet more fully myself.

I arrived finally into a world of therapeutic insight and intersubjectivity, where Bromberg might say I could "stand in the spaces," Richard Geist could show me the internal spaces of therapeutic connectedness, in which "connectedness refers …

DOI: 10.4324/9781003340751-14

to a consciously or non-consciously felt sense of sharing and participating in another's subjective emotional life, while simultaneously experiencing another as participating in one's own subjective life" (p. 134), all of which I discovered in my own analysis with Ernest S. Wolf.

All along the way, I read and studied the literature and culture of the ancient Greeks, where I found an archaic psyche open to gods, nature, and community – a polytheistic culture that seemed not yet to have formed an internalized psyche with its own agency and political nature in the Greek civic state of 5th century BCE Athens. This Classical psyche developed from a newly found freedom, less dependent on the gods and a powerfully ritualized mother nature. The Classical psyche reveled in its newfound independence, relying on its own patriarchal autocracy. The earlier Homeric *Iliad*, an epic of heroic emphasis on grandeur and glory, and the ancient Greek tragedies that blossomed in Classical Athens following it, convinced me of how disastrous the suppression of matricentric values were to this early western culture, and how deeply our present psychotherapeutic practices are redemptive for us in their intersubjective and maternal approaches to healing.

I realize now that I have been on an Odyssean journey to find a home where male and female values can exist together in an equality of strength, intelligence, and compassion. Odysseus and Penelope, two tricksters of equal intelligence and resilience, join together at last when Penelope slyly asks Odysseus to move their marriage bed, and Odysseus says he cannot, because he built it such that one of its legs is a tree trunk. Penelope recognizes at that moment that this now old man that she hasn't seen for 20 years is indeed her husband. In their intimate joining, I think of intimate moments of being in the therapy room where therapist and patient come fully together in transcendent space. These moments are ineffable. They feel like transformative unions, or what Jung calls the "coniunctio," a mystical union where through metaphorical alchemical processes, analyst, and analysand come into an embodied yet disembodied wholeness (C.G. Jung, 1966a, p. 169, paras. 354 ff). It is here that one discovers that individuation is what leads to a sense of transfiguration and the divine, where the universal and the particular become one.

Both Liza and Amanda underwent metamorphoses, Liza from a cocooned traumatized woman to a soaring butterfly, and Amanda from a glowing, exquisite, and magnificent performer shattered by childhood trauma and deadly disease to a hawk that could fly free. Immersing myself empathically in their own images and believing that the images themselves had the transformative power to heal convinced me that staying with the language of myths of metamorphoses might better aid their healing process than the diagnostic categories in which I had been trained.

These patients transformed the consulting room for me into a force field in which new, aesthetic realms of experience and meaning flowing with vivid symbols, images and dreams could become genuinely existent for them as they became so for me. Therapy resembled a kind of transubstantiation – an invitation for me to be caught up with them in liminal spaces fervently alive with vibrant and creative energy. Both Amanda and Liza accomplished this by trustfully allowing themselves to be held by what had been for them a lost realm of the maternal, a realm of birthing and dying and rebirth, ending in *autopoiesis*, a space of self-creation.

I began to muse further on whether what we call borderline personalities today might be better understood as subjects of living metamorphoses. Could we perhaps call every psyche graced with a well-circumscribed western ego one prone to borderline phenomena of one sort or another? Descartes himself held that we should allow nothing into our minds except clear and distinct ideas or those that can be deduced from these axioms. For him the only way to think about nature clearly and distinctly is through mathematics. Symbols, images, colors, diaphanous presences, liminal and imaginal spaces are all now cast out of experience and pure, logical rationality reigns supreme. Heidegger talks about dwelling with the divinities, trying to find a way of being in the world not conceptualized by our ideas, but in which we are together with earth, sky, mortals, and immortals, that is, with the being of the world, rather than a world organized through our concepts.

Heidegger and my own experiences with the liminality that I inhabited with my two early patients brought me back to the mythic imagination of Ovid's *Metamorphoses*, psychologically so meaningful in their expression of the shifts and changes of our being and how we might live with nature, the divine, and others in ourselves. This in turn reminded me of what Bromberg (1998) calls an existence rich with multiple, yet still dissociated self states.

11.1.1 Ovid's Metamorphoses and Clinical Diagnoses

Ovid's rendition of Greek myths highlights the borders between the animate and inanimate, human and non-human, where identities are transformed in perhaps needed and positive ways that seem like punishment only to an ego certain of its human infallibility. These thoughts further convinced me that in working with clinically diagnosable narcissism like Amanda's, it was more meaningful to speak in this liminal, symbolic language, where, for example, the being of a diagnosed borderline personality might be better felt through transformative and poetic descriptions of myths of metamorphosis, and where specific kinds of soul landscapes are understood as a part of a coherent, although multiple wholeness.

Perhaps such permutations and combinations are necessary for feeling united with nature and the divine. Why, for example, is it a punishment for Daphne to be turned into a tree? Or Io, into a cow? The anthropomorphism of the ancient Greek cosmos might reveal a longing for reconnection with a sense of the sacredness of nature that we have lost and long to reintegrate. If the laurel wreath with which Apollo crowned his poets and victors had not been formed from the laurel tree that was formerly a living nymph whose father was a river, so much a part of nature, would it have been so special? In reading the *Metamorphoses*, I could imagine that what we might think of clinically as a breakdown was simultaneously a "breakthrough" (Field, 1996, p. 12), precisely because in reading these myths we are lured into loosening our own ego boundaries to reimagine supposed pathologies as symbolic landscapes and stories creating fresh, vital therapeutic space. I began to wonder whether musing on revisioning our clinical diagnoses might lead us into a new kind of therapeutic space that could in turn lead us to imagining a new kind of psyche, simultaneously more inclusive and more mutable.

Amanda, for example, as a divine, idealizable narcissist, is like Ovid's Narcissus (who is not quite the figure that Freud or Kohut make him out to be, although he is much closer to Kohut's understanding). The myth itself tells of a young man who falls in love with his own reflection in a pond and is so in love that he merges with it, transforming into a beautiful flower with an impossibly sweet, drug-inducing scent, still called a narcissus today.

In a part of this myth that we don't ordinarily hear about, Liriope and Cephisus, Narcissus' parents, are water nymphs, ever undefined, ever flowing and changing, able only to be rippling mirrors for their longing son. When Liriope asks Tiresias, the prophet, if Narcissus will have a long life, he answers that he will, "unless he comes to recognize himself." What a strange statement, and what a strange question for a mother to ask! Perhaps it means that in Narcissus' coming to love his own reflection he will find out his background and, consequently, who he really is. Because of his parents, a watery reflection is perhaps closer to a more authentic state for him than his own fleshly embodiment. Or, perhaps, there is a warning here about "coming to know himself" in a way that will remove him from the nature of which he has always been an integral part.

What Kohut might call Narcissus' narcissistic grandeur can be understood partly in mythic terms as his inevitable abandonment at birth, given that his parents were disembodied. Narcissus' wish, to possess his own watery reflection as a lover, is tragic (rather than pathological) because it represents his sense of emotional emptiness, loss, and abandonment at having had to give up a watery sphere which was his birthright. If he is to relate to his mother, he must return to her watery womb. The tragedy for Narcissus may be that he is too caught up in the absence of his parents ever to engage in mortal, substantial union. He spends his life scarcely born, in a still, pure, unchanging forest.

A Kohutian perspective might suggest that this myth shows us that Narcissus experiences sufficiently severe "narcissistic" injury in his inevitable parental abandonment that he is too wounded ever to develop selfobject relationships. He falls in love with his own reflection wavering and shifting in the water in a desperate attempt to create himself. Even the nymph Echo, who loves him hopelessly, can only exist as Narcissus' own echo. At the end of Ovid's myth, Narcissus mourns just as Echo did at its start, a bodyless and yearning flame:

> Secretly she glided
> Fired with love to follow him; and as she
> came closer to his side, the very source
> Of flames increased her heat; she was as sulphur
> at the tip of torches, leaping to fire
> When another flame leans towards it.
> (Ovid, *Metamorphoses*, 1958, p. 96 [*Met. III*, 370–373])

Amanda's birthright was not unlike this. It was itself absent of the secure and trustworthy selfobject relationships that her parents could have been for her, and the absence, longing, and despair created in this myth is also what Amanda feels as she takes leave of her body in her passage to death. She mourns a life heroically lived in finding herself reflected through me, her therapist, as a rippling mirror before she takes leave of life. It is this kind of mythic telling and musing on the nature of metamorphosis that can transform the therapy room into a vivid, alive, aesthetic space that can create healing, but can also dissolve into a watery and dangerous kind of vulnerability, if the believing therapist is not present as a holding container.

In this gathering of mythically aesthetic forms of transformation in the therapy room, I am also aware of how Jungians work through dreams, archetypes, and stories. And I feel ever more strongly that healing is achieved through living in and with symbols that transform, because it is these in particular that engage the analytic dyad in relationship through their affective power. It is this language that ultimately brings the self to feel at home in the relationship, whether living a healthy narcissistic life or, as in treating Amanda, finding a safe home as she moves through the end of her life into death. It is especially in the third fields that exist between us and surround us that this kind of language is birthed and carries meanings that heal. "Kohut's self is an open system not delimited by physical boundaries" (Ornstein, 1980). Therefore, there is an inherent metaphorical fluidity to interacting "selfs," which is heuristically suggestive of a shared and overlapping emotional life regardless of how much asymmetry we attribute to the analytic dyad (Geist, 2008, p. 135).

It would have been futile to engage other clinical approaches to try to help Amanda. She wanted neither earth nor Olympus, but to be held in this space between, this liminal space between life and death where one yearns to drift without limits and to be free of mortal pain. This is the space that I needed to hold and contain without pulling her back to an earthly possibility for coherence that had perhaps never been possible for her. I recognized through Amanda that living on the borders of the space of the daemonic and being seen as part of that mythic landscape, aesthetic language can be honored and reflected in such a way as to bring integrity and acceptance to the tragedy and fallibility of our humanness.

Amanda's and Liza's stories are important because they show an isolation redeemed through dwelling in the liminal. Amanda is willing to reveal to me her own capacity for imaginative creation before she discards it. Yet both women tell me that there is a world of imaginal dwelling in which they can feel free. I would like to think that perhaps they could do so because I was able to hold this aesthetic space with them.

Most of us need to move into transitional experience from a state of fusion with our caretakers because we feel the need to adventure into the creativity of being our own subjects apart from them. Amanda had never had the luxury of being part of a mother/baby unit, but found it, perhaps with my containment, in the energy field itself which, after all, had become her new home. Perhaps in the cases of both Liza end Amanda, staying consistently with them through the discovery of their aesthetic, imaginative experiences helped them, each in their own way, to find a therapeutic cradle of trust that promises integration and freedom.

11.1.2 C.G. Jung's Coniunctio

Liza's and Amanda's cases both suggest that the achievement of a sense of multiple coherence needs to occur in a place of coupling with a good-enough mother therapist. The *coniunctio*, or unconscious, mystical union felt between therapist and patient can then help the patient to couple with herself in such a way that she can sense herself as a self in union with her inner and outer psychic realms. The archaic Greek psyche also depicts this ultimate *coniunctio*. It happens in moments of understanding that self-coherence is found by returning to one's connection with an archaic and archetypal maternal world, as did Odysseus and Penelope.

Exploring this notion of *coniunctio* leads to a vital mythic space, and shows us that this connection can be found through the acceptance of mortality as it opens the psyche into the possibility of a return to the mother, even and perhaps especially in the process of individuation, as Jung and Schwartz-Salant describe it. *Indeed, individuation presupposes interconnection, bonding, and webbing*.

We see this kind of union in Oedipus at the end of the *Oedipus at Colonus*, and at the end of the story of the life of Pentheus and Thebes as described by Ovid, in reference to Pentheus' grandparents, Cadmus and Harmonia. In the *Oedipus at Colonus* Sophocles (1973) R. Fitzgerald, trans.) we meet blind, old Oedipus leaning on his daughter for support, fully dependent on her for his sight. Suffering and long years, he says, have taught him contentment. In this final drama about Oedipus, words describing non-sexual love (*philia, storge*) take precedence over the word eros, or sexual love. Oedipus is able now to recognize that he is innocent of the crimes against his parents. In the context of destiny and the content of his acts, however, he takes responsibility for what he has done. He knows, too, that this destiny will have him enter the grove of the Eumenides and become a blessing for Athens through his own burial.

Yet Oedipus is still Oedipus. Although he is no longer sleeping with his personal mother, his destiny compels him to enter the secret and untouchable grove of the Eumenides which is referred to in the drama as the sacred place of Dionysus, of Aphrodite, and of Demeter and Persephone:

> Here with drops of heaven's dews
> at daybreak all the year,
> The clusters of narcissus bloom,
> Time-hallowed garlands for the brows
> Of those great ladies whom we fear.
>
> The crocus like a little sun
> blooms with its yellow ray;
> the river's fountains are awake,
> and his nomadic streams that run
> unthinned forever, and never stay;
>
> But like perpetual lovers move
> on the maternal land.
> And here the choiring Muses come,
> And the divinity of love
> with the gold reins in her hand.
>
> (Soph. *OC* ll. 681–695, trans. R. Fitzgerald, 1973)

At the end of Oedipus' life, a lightning strike splits open the earth, and in this symbolic and cosmic reminiscence of his own act of intercourse with his mother, he is taken again back into his mother, only this time it is Gaia, Mother Earth, herself. This move from the personal and unconscious act to the symbolic, archetypal act brings Oedipus to recognition of his true identity. He understands that his attainment of divinity in blessing happens only in the context of his dependence upon destiny in the season's cycles. There is a sense now that he is living in an interconnected way, still like a lover, with the maternal cosmos that gives him and others strength and blessing in his particular identity. This happens only at his death. But is it not possible that in the telling of this death, Sophocles, at his own age of 92, is telling us about an ultimate individuation in the recognition of one's own deep bonds with the maternal cosmos (Dobson, 2007)?

In Euripides' *Bacchae* (1958) (H. Gregory, trans.), Cadmus and Harmonia, because of the crime of their daughter Agave's slaughter of their grandchild, Pentheus, are compelled to fulfill an oracle: they are turned to serpents and, pulling a chariot, they leave the destroyed Thebes to enter the lands of a blessed and divine nature. Ovid tells this story in such a way as to suggest that the acceptance of oneself as a part of a cosmic nature after the struggle to attain ego can bring interconnectedness without fear.

In Ovid's telling of the myth, Cadmus asks if it was perchance his own stabbing of the holy serpent for the purpose of founding Thebes that caused his disowning by the gods. He asks if he might become a serpent, in retribution for his sins:

> He grew reptilian features everywhere:
> His skin turned hard and scales swarmed over it
> And shining spots glittered across his body;
> He fell flat downward to the earth – his legs
> A tail that whipped the ground beneath it.
> (Ovid, 1958, p. 129 [*Met. IV*, 576–579])

Here is a man who accepts his mortality fully, as well as the fate that has come of his trying to found a city and move away from a seemingly uncontrollable mother nature. Aged and experienced, he calls out to his beloved wife to come near him, "While something of myself is left to call you/Before the serpent swallows all of me/Touch me and hold my hand within your hand" (p. 129 [*Met. IV*, 584–585]). Cadmus asks for connection, and his queen comes to him at first as human:

> He glided from her girdle to her throat
> Those who looked on and saw them as they were
> … grew terrified -
> And yet their queen caressed the plumed snake
> They looked again and saw them as in bed
> Their bodies joined as in a last embrace.
> (p. 129 [*Met. IV*, 595–599])

Cadmus and Harmonia breathe the tragic quality of acceptance of the fall from mortality as recompense for the obsessive misogynism of the hubristic ruler, their grandson Pentheus, who represses his own sexual and aggressive impulses and, in so doing, rejects the maternal feminine. The result is that his own mother decapitates him thinking that he is a lion. Cadmus and Harmonia in their own lives experience the perfect union that leads to an acceptance of the world as it is in its multiplicity of metamorphoses. This *coniunctio*, which for Jung is not just a union, but a "mystical marriage" (Jung, 1966a, Vol. XVI, p. 169: para. 355), arises out of caring and tending the otherness that each is in their sameness:

> And yet, a moment after this, two serpents
> were seen that vanished deep in the green forest
> Who neither feared nor fought with anyone,
> Calm dragons that had cherished what they were.
> (p. 129 [Ovid, *Met. IV*, 600–601])

In Euripides' *Bacchae* (1954), we understand once again, as Aristotle says, that the real meaning of tragedy comes in the recognition of the *hamartia*, or "tragic flaw" of the protagonist, which seems in drama after drama to be the inevitability of mortality itself. The stories of old Oedipus, and Cadmus and Harmonia remind us how important it is, if we are to have a full and realized life, to learn how to yield ourselves compassionately to relationships and to an acceptance of nature, the divine and others of our own species.

In the moments of transitional experiencing in psychotherapy, where borders are fluid, it is the interactive, imaginal field that makes possible containment and coherence. It is the therapist, empathizing deeply with the sufferer whose spirit is caught powerfully in the earthly soul it both longs to escape from and to be substantiated by, who invites the living symbolic experience that can birth the multiply coherent psyche. In mythic landscapes, words like "borderline" and "narcissist" melt into colors and shapes that undergo metamorphosis or transformation simply by being held by the poet, or the therapist who is there to listen to the hearkening of the psyche of her patient and herself as they experience together their freedoms and the vicissitudes of intersubjectivity. Poet and therapist alike tell us that the return to nature as maternal is crucial, the maternal that was shunned and repressed by a western, androcentric ego structure, which needed to contain itself rigidly to feel safe in a new civic world.

This is a realm that speaks the language of spirit and soul, not just pathology and symptom. It is here that we, as therapists and poets, can understand the plenitude of the world we inhabit and have faith in our calling.

References

Bollas, C. (1987). *The Shadow of the Object: Psychoanalysis of the Unthought Known.* New York: Columbia University Press.

Bromberg, P. (1998). *Standing in the Spaces: Essays on Clinical Process, Trauma and Dissociation* (1st ed.). London: Psychology Press.

Dobson, M.W. D-S. Freud, Kohut, Sophocles: Did Oedipus do wrong? *International Journal of Self Psychology*, 2(1) 2007.

Euripides (1954). *The Bacchae and Other Plays* (P. Vellacott, trans.). New York: Viking Penguin.

Field, N. (1996). *Breakdown and Breakthrough: Psychotherapy in a New Dimension.* New York: Routledge.

Geist, R.A. (2008) Connectedness, permeable boundaries, and the development of the self: Therapeutic Implications. *International Journal of Psychoanalytic Self Psychology* 3: 129–152.

Jung, C.G. (1966a). The psychology of the transference. In R.F.C. Hull (trans.), *The Collected Works of C.G. Jung* (Vol. 16). (2nd ed.). Princeton: Princeton University Press. (Original work published in 1954.)

Ornstein, P.H. (1980). Self-psychology and the concept of health. In A. Goldberg (ed.), *Advances* in *Self Psychology.* New York: International Universities Press.

Ovid (1958). *The Metamorphoses.* (H. Gregory, trans.). New York: Viking Press.

Sophocles (1973). *Sophocles I: Oedipus* the *King* (D. Grene, trans.) *Oedipus at Colonus* (R. Fitzgerald, trans.), *Antigone* (E. Wyckoff, trans.). Chicago: University of Chicago.

Chapter 12

Concluding Thoughts

In this book, I have considered 1) various theories of transitional, and transformational space as understood by psychoanalytic theorists, 2) my own personal experience as both a patient and a psychoanalytically attuned relational self psychologist, and 3) languages of liminal space through an imaginative inquiry into the movement of the pre-platonic archaic and permeable psyche of the ancient Greeks as seen through a few of the works of their major authors, to the formation of a more bounded western ego that now has to transform, once again, to be effective in our more complex and suffering world. I hope I have been persuasive in showing that living always in the atmosphere of paradoxes of the transitional and transformational presents us with the possibility of accepting "otherness" in ourselves as well as in others, delighting in the permeable boundaries among humans as well as the mysteries of nature and community surrounding us and within us. This is a space where we can discover profound aesthetic and emotional nourishment. This is also a space where we can be safely cradled, returning to an inevitably lost maternal connection through our own aesthetic creations.

The ancient Greek authors that I have considered move us into an aestheticization of intermediate space, which allows us to return to the world from which we feel acutely our separation and desire to regain connection. Art itself becomes a transitional field through its aesthetic languages of culture and self through which we can recuperate our maternal idiom and dare to dive into those tremulous spaces of the "unknown," and "sort of known" (Bromberg, 2010), to allow a newly created, harmonious

DOI: 10.4324/9781003340751-15

form of interweaving that permits us to gain rather than to lose ourselves. In fact, it is in the very process of finding a robust self through creativity that enhances relationship and intersubjectivity and that allows us to live without fear of dissolution. Recognition of liminal experience and dwelling in it connects us with the feminine/maternal – the personal as well as the cultural mother – whose loss we most especially grieve. That grief opens us to the possibility of recuperating "mother" and the maternal idiom through our own creations.

The ancient Greeks expressed this sense of loss not only through a new kind of writing, but through archetypal stories that became personally and culturally idiosyncratic in their myths. Stories and myths of lost homes and lost paradises abound, yet Pygmalian must create his own statue of the perfect woman that perfectly mirrors him and long for her to come to life to be his wife, because he can no longer stand the animalistic, orgiastic rituals of the goddess Aphrodite. More subjectivity is needed. Orpheus in the beauty of his music expressing the loss of his Eurydice can touch Nature herself. Through the sounds of his lyre, he makes stones hurled at him by the maenads stop in their tracks in the air and weep under the earth at his death. Even Persephone, the dark, dread queen of the underworld, weeps and relents when she hears his music, promising to send Eurydice back to the living world. Such is the power of art and longing to recuperate the mother and to transform nature.

The loss of the great maternal as we separate from the earth to develop self-consciousness is equivalent to the loss of the personal mother. It is through the inevitable loss of the maternal that we gain perspective. As we perceive the mother as object, we know that we are no longer of her, but have separated. It is this sense of both loneliness and freedom that creates a transitional, transformative field that we can hover and be nested in and in which we can learn to hold ourselves strong. That same strength is needed to then be in deep intersubjective community with others. If we are the eyes of nature, and this very development of perspective "others" us, then part of us lives in mourning and longs to return to what we have lost. We feel the imperative need to join with it again through our own "aesthetic resonances" and creative reformulations (Hagman, 2010, p. 192) This creative reformulation becomes itself a subjective object to the artist, who molds and crafts it such that it stands as his own but also as a mixture of himself with the community (pp. 31–32). Engaging creatively in this way with otherness and others provides consolation and possibility for redeeming a chaotic and destructive world.

References

Bromberg, P. (2010). *Knowing, Not Knowing, and Sort of Knowing.* London. Routledge.

Hagman, G. (2010). *The Artist's Mind: Art Creativity and Clinical Process.* London. Routledge.

Bibliography

Aeschyli (1964). *Septem quae supersunt tragoediae* (The seven remaining tragedies). G. Murray (ed.). London: Oxford University Press.

Aeschylus (1979). *The Oresteia* (H. Lloyd Jones, trans.). Berkeley, CA: University of California Press.

Alford, C.F. (1992). *The Psychoanalytic Theory of Greek Tragedy.* New Haven, CT: Yale University Press.

American Psychiatric Association (1994). *Diagnostic and Statistical Manual of Mental Disorders* (4th ed.). Washington, DC: Author.

Aristotle (1983). Poetics. In H.G. Apostle and L.P. Gerson (trans.), *Aristotle: Selected Works* (pp. 645–681). Grinnell, IA: Peripatetic Press.

Atwood, G.E. (2012). *The Abyss of Madness.* London: Routledge.

Bacal, H.A. (1989). Winnicott and self-psychology: Remarkable reflections. In D.W. and S.P. Detrick, *Self-psychology: Comparisons and Contrasts* (pp. 259–274). Hillsdale, NJ: Analytic Press.

Bacal, H.A. (1990). The elements of a corrective self object experience. *Psychoanalytic Inquiry*, 10(3): 347–372.

Bachofen, J.J. (1967). *Myth, Religion, & Mother Right: Selected Writings of J.J. Bachofen* (R. Mannheim, trans.) Princeton, NJ: Princeton University Press.

Bakker, E. (1997). Storytelling in the future: Truth, time and tense in Homeric epic. In E. Bakker and A. Kahane (eds.), *Written Voices, Spoken Signs: Tradition, Performance, and the Epic* (pp. 11–37). Cambridge, MA: Harvard University Press.

Barnes, H.E. (1974). *The Meddling Gods: Four Essays on Classical Themes.* Lincoln: University of Nebraska Press.

Bergman, A. (1995). From mother to the world outside: The use of space during the separation-individuation phase. In S.A. Grolnick and L. Barkin (eds.), *Between Reality and Fantasy. Winnicott's Concepts of Transitional Objects and Phenomena* (pp. 145–167). Northvale, NJ: Jason Aronson, Inc.

Boedeker, D. (1984). *Descent from Heaven: Images of Dew in Greek Poetry and Religion.* Chico, CA: Scholar Press.

Bohm, D. (1980). *Wholeness and the Implicate Order.* London: Routledge.

Bollas, C. (1987). *The Shadow of the Object: Psychoanalysis of the Unthought Known.* New York: Columbia University Press.

Bowlby, J. (1969). *Attachment and Loss* (Vol. 1). New York: Basic Books.

Briffault, R. (1977). *The Mothers.* New York: Atheneum.

Bronstein, A.A. (1992). The fetish, transitional objects, and illusion. *Psychoanalytic Review*, 79(2): 239–260.

Bromberg, P. (1998). *Standing in the Spaces: Essays on Clinical Process, Trauma and Dissociation* (1st ed.). London: Psychology Press.

Bromberg, P. (2010). *Knowing, Not Knowing, and Sort of Knowing.* London: Routledge.

Burkert, W. (1985). *Greek Religion.* London: Basil Blackwell.

Butterworth, E.A.S. (1970). *The Tree at the Navel of the Earth.* Berlin: De Gruyter.

Caldwell, R. (1985). The power of Aphrodite: Eros and the boundaries of the self in the *Hippolytus.* In P. Burian (ed.), *Directions in Euripidean Criticism* (pp. 52–110). Durham, NC: Duke University Press.

Campbell, J. (ed.) (1971). *The Portable Jung* (R.F.C. Hull, trans.). New York: Penguin Books.

Charlton, R.S. (1997). Fictions of the internal object. *Journal of Analytical Psychology*, 42: 81–99.

Chodorow, N. (1978). *The Reproduction of Mothering.* Berkeley: University of California Press.

Cixous, H. (1994). The laugh of the Medusa. In Susan Sellers et al. (eds.), *The Helene Cixous Reader*. London: Routledge.

Coburn, W.J. (2013). *Psychoanalytic Complexity: Clinical Attitudes for Therapeutic Change* (Psychoanalytic Inquiry Book Series). London: Routledge.

Cohler, B.J. (1980). Developmental perspectives on the psychology of the self in early childhood. In A. Goldberg (ed.), *Advances in Self Psychology* (pp. 69–115). New York: International Universities Press, Inc.

Cornford, F. (1912). *From Religion to Philosophy.* London: Arnold.

Descartes, R. (1979). *Meditations on First Philosophy.* (D.A. Cress, trans.). Indianapolis: Hackett Publishing Co.

Detienne, M. (1986). *The Creation of Mythology*. (M. Cook, trans.). Chicago: University of Chicago Press.

Detienne, M. (1996). *The Masters of Truth in Archaic Greece.* (J. Lloyd, trans.). New York: Urzone, Inc.

Devereux, G. (1985). *The Character of the Euripidean Hippolytos: An Ethno-psychoanalytical Study.* Chico, CA: Scholar Press.

Diels, H. and Kranz, W. (eds.) (1954). *Die Fragmente der Vorsokratilcer* (The fragments of the Presocratics) (6th ed.). Berlin: Weidmannsche Buchhandlung.

Dobson, M. (2018). Why Does Orestes Stay Mad? in J. Lauwers, H. Schwall, and J. Opsomer (eds.), *Psychology and the Classics: A Dialogue of Disciplines* (pp. 158–170). Berlin: De Gruyter.

Dobson, M.D.-S. (2020). Young Kohut and the ancient Greek satyr play. *Psychoanalysis, Self and Context*, 15(1).

Dobson, M. D-S. (2018). Weaving the dream fields of Jung and Kohut. In R.S. Brown (ed.), *Re-Encountering Jung: Analytical Psychology and Contemporary Psychoanalysis*. London. Routledge.

Dobson, M. (2015). Transcendent dimensions of the self: A spiritual home for self psychology? *International Journal of Psychoanalytic Self Psychology*, 10(1): 1–13.

Dobson, M.W.D-S. (2007). Freud, Kohut, Sophocles: Did Oedipus do wrong? *International Journal of Self Psychology*, 2: 1.

Dobson, M.W.D-S. (1984, July). Unpublished Journal.

Dobson, M.W.D-S. and Riker, J. (1976–97). "Greek History and Philosophy." Colorado Springs: Colorado College.

Dodds, E.R. (1951). *The Greeks and the Irrational.* Berkeley: University of California Press.

Dodds, E.R. (ed.). (1974). *Euripides' Bacchae.* London: Clarendon Press.

Downing, C. (ed.). (1994). *The Long Journey Home: Revisioning the Myth of Demeter and Persephone for Our Time.* Boston, MA: Shambhala.

DuBois, P. (1986). *Sowing the Body: Psychoanalysis and Ancient Representations of Women.* Chicago: University of Chicago Press.

Dunbar, H.F. (1929). *Symbolism in Medieval Thought and its Consummation in the Divine Comedy*. New Haven: Yale University Press.

Dunbar, F. (1954). *Emotions and Bodily Changes: A survey of literature on psychosomatic interrelationships, 1910–1953* (3rd ed.). NY: Columbia University Press.

Eigen, M. (1981). The area of faith in Winnicott, Lacan and Bion. *International Journal of Psychoanalysis*, 62: 413–433.
Eigen, M. (1996). *Psychic Deadness.* Northvale, NJ: Jason Aronson.
Eisler, R. (1987). *The Chalice and the Blade: Our History, Our Future.* San Francisco, CA: Harper & Row.
Eshel, O. (2006). Where are you, my beloved? *International Journal of Psychoanalysis*, 87(6): 1603–1627.
Euripides (1954). *The Bacchae and Other Plays* (P. Vellacott, trans.). New York: Viking Penguin, Inc.
Farnell, L.R. (1896–1909). *The Cults of the Greek States* (Vols. 1–5). London: Oxford University Press.
Field, N. (1996). *Breakdown and Breakthrough: Psychotherapy in a New Dimension.* New York: Routledge.
Foley, H.P. (ed.). (1994). *The Homeric Hymn to Demeter: Translation, Commentary and Interpretive Essays.* Princeton, NJ: Princeton University Press.
Frame, D. (1978). *The Myth of Return in Early Greek Epic.* New Haven, CT: Yale University Press.
Frazer, J.G. (1911–1915). *The Golden Bough: A Study in Magic and Religion* (Vols. 1–12). London: McMillan & Co.
Freud, S. (1917). Mourning and melancholia. Vol. 14, p. 239 of *The Standard Edition of the complete works of Sigmund Freud* (J. Strachey, trans.). London: Hogarth Press (1953–74).
Freud, S. (1915). The unconscious. Vol. 14, p. 161 of *The Standard Edition of the complete works of Sigmund Freud* (J. Strachey, trans.). London: Hogarth Press (1953–74).
Gilligan, C. (1982). *In a Different Voice: Psychological Theory and Women's Development*. Cambridge: Harvard University Press.
Gimbutas, M. (1989). *The Language of the Goddess*. San Francisco: Harper and Row.
Golden, G.K. and Hill, M.A. (1991). A token of loving: From melancholia to mourning. *Clinical Social Work Journal*, 19: 23–33.
Goldhill, S. (1986). *Reading Greek Tragedy.* Cambridge, UK: Cambridge University Press.
Goodison, L. (1989). *Death, Women and the Sun.* BICS Supplement #530. London.
Gouldner, A. (1965). *Enter Plato*. New York: Basic Books.
Green, A. (1975). The analyst, symbolization, and absence in the analytic setting. *International Journal of Psycho-Analysis*, 56: 1–22.
Greenberg, J.R. and Mitchell, S.A. (1983). *Object Relations in Psychoanalytic Theory.* Cambridge, MA: Harvard University Press.

Grolnick, S.A. (1995). Dreams and dreaming as transitional phenomena. In S.A. Grolnick and L. Barkin (eds.), *Between Reality and Fantasy: Winnicott's Concepts of Transitional Objects and Phenomena* (pp. 245–257). Northvale, NJ: Jason Aronson, Inc.

Grotstein, J. (1993). *Splitting and Projective Identification.* Northvale, NJ: Jason Aronson, Inc.

Grotstein, J. (1997). Internal objects or chimerical monsters. *Journal of Analytical Psychology*, 42: 45–80.

Hagman, G. (2016). New mourning: A new psychoanalytic understanding and treatment of mourning. In G. Hagman (ed.), *New Models of Bereavement Theory and Treatment: New Mourning* (Ch. 12). London: Routledge.

Hagman, G. (2015). *Creative Analysis: Art, Creativity and Clinical Process.* London: Routledge.

Hagman, G. (2011). *Aesthetic Experience: Beauty, Creativity, and the Search for the Ideal.* Amsterdam: Rodopi.

Hagman, G. (2010). *The Artist's Mind: Art Creativity and Clinical Process.* London: Routledge.

Hagman, G. (2001). Beyond decathexis: Towards a new psychoanalytic understanding and treatment of mourning. In R. Neimeyer (ed.), *Meaning, Reconstruction and the Experience of Loss.* New York: American Psychological Association.

Harrison, J.E. (1962a). *Epilegomena to the Study of Greek religion and Themis: A Study of the Social Origins of Greek Religion.* New York: University Books.

Harrison, J.E. (1962b). *Themis: A Study of the Social Origins of Greek Religion.* Cleveland: Meridian Press.

Heidegger, M. (1971). Building, dwelling, thinking. In J. Hofstadter (trans.), *Poetry, Language, Thought* (pp. 143–162). New York: Harper Colophon.

Herodotus (1972). *The Histories* (A. de Selincourt, trans.). Baltimore: Penguin.

Hesiod (1920). *Hesiod, the Homeric Hymns and Homerica* (H.G. Evelyn-White, ed. and trans.). London: William Heinemann.

Hillman, J. (1975). *Revisioning Psychology.* New York: Harper Colophon.

Hillman, J. (1983). *Archetypal Psychology.* Dallas, TX: Spring Publications.

Hillman, J. (1993). *Suicide and the Soul.* Dallas, TX: Spring Publications.

Homer (1990). *The Iliad* (R. Fagles, trans.). New York: Viking Penguin.

Homer (1996). *The Odyssey* (R. Fagles, trans.). New York: Penguin Putnam.

Homeric Hymn to Demeter (1920). *Hesiod, The Homeric Hymns and Homerica* (H.G. Evelyn White, trans.). Cambridge, MA: Harvard University Press.

Jaynes, J. (1976). *The Origins of Consciousness in the Breakdown of the Bicameral Mind.* Boston: Houghton Mifflin Company.

Jordan, J.V., Surrey, J.L. and Kaplan, A.G. (1991). Women and empathy: Implications for psychological development and psychotherapy. In *Women's Growth in Connection* (pp. 27–50). New York: Guilford Press.

Jung, C.G. (1965). *Memories, Dreams, Reflections.* New York: Random House.

Jung, C.G. (1966). The Philosophical Tree, Para. 482, pp. 348–349. In R.F.C. Hull (trans.), *The Collected Works of C.G. Jung* (Vol. 13) (2nd ed.). Princeton: Princeton University Press. (Original work published in 1954).

Jung, C.G. (1966b). The psychology of the transference. In R.F.C. Hull (trans.), *The Collected Works of C.G. Jung* (Vol. 16) (2nd ed.). Princeton, NJ: Princeton University Press. (Original work published in 1954.)

Jung, C.G. (1969). The archetypes and the collective unconscious. In R.F.C. Hull (trans.). *The Collected Works of C.G. Jung* (Vol. IX) (2nd ed). Princeton, NJ: Princeton University Press. (Original work published in 1959.)

Jung, C.G. (1978). Alon. In R.F.C. Hull (trans.), *The Collected Works of C.G. Jung* (Vol 9ii) (2nd ed.). Princeton, NJ: Princeton University Press. (Original work published in 1951.)

Jung, C.G. (1980). Psychology and alchemy. In R.F.C. Hull (trans.), *The Collected Works of C.G. Jung* (Vol. 12). Princeton, NJ: Princeton University Press. (Original work published in 1953.)

Jung, C.G. (1981). On the nature of the psyche. In R.F.C. Hull (trans.). *The Collected Works of C.G. Jung* (Vol. 8) (2nd ed.) Princeton, NJ: Princeton University Press. (Original work published in 1960.)

Jung, C.G. (1989). Mysterium coniunctionis. In R.F.C. Hull (trans.), *The Collected Works of C.G. Jung* (Vol. 14). Princeton, NJ: Princeton University Press. (Original work published in 1955.)

Jung, C.G. (2008). *The Earth Has a Soul: C.G. Jung on Nature, Technology and Modern Life.* (M. Sabini, ed.) Berkeley, CA: North Atlantic Press.

Jung, C.G. and Kerenyi, C. (1963). *Essays on a Science of Mythology: The Myth of the Divine Child and the Mysteries of Eleusis* (1973). Princeton, NJ: New Jersey, Princeton University Press.

Kahn, C.H. (1979). *The Art and Thought of Heraclitus: An Edition of the Fragments with Translation and Commentary*. Cambridge, UK: Cambridge University Press.

Kalsched, D. (2013). *Trauma and the Soul: A Psycho-spiritual Approach to Human Development and its Interruption*. London: Routledge.

Keller, C. (1986). *From a Broken Web: Separatism, Sexism, and Self.* Boston, MA: Beacon Press.

Kerenyi, C. (1967). *Eleusis: Archetypal Image of Mother and Daughter* (R. Manheim, trans.) Princeton, NJ: Princeton University Press. (Original work published in 1960.)

Klein, M. (1963). Some reflections on Aeschylus' *Oresteia*. In *Envy and Gratitude and Other Works* (pp. 275–299). New York: Free Press. (Original work published in 1940.)

Klein, M. (1964). Mourning and its relation to manicdepressive states. In M. Klein (ed.), *Contributions to Psycho-analysis 1921–1945* (pp. 311–338). New York: McGraw-Hill Book Company. (Original work published in 1940.)

Kohut, H. (1966). Forms and transformations of Narcissism. *Journal of the American Psychoanalytic Association*, 14: 243–272.

Kohut, H. (1971). *The Analysis of the Self: A Systematic Approach to the Psychoanalytic Treatment of Narcissistic Personality Disorders*. New York: International Universities Press, Inc.

Kohut, H. (1977). *The Restoration of the Self.* New York: International Universities Press.

Kohut, H. (1984). *How Does Analysis Cure*? (A. Goldberg and P. Stepansky, eds.). Chicago: Chicago University Press.

Kohut, H. (1991). Kohut and the search for the self. Vol. 4. In P. Ornstein (ed.), *Introspection, Empathy and the Semi-circle of Mental Health* (pp. 537–567). Madison, CT: International University Press.

Kulka, R. (2012). Between emergence and dissolving: Contemporary reflections on greatness and ideals in Kohut's legacy. *International Journal of Psychoanalytic Self Psychology*, 7(2): 264–285.

Kulka, R. (2021). Self psychology: The ethics of oneness. *Psychoanalytic Review*, 108: 141–153.

Linker, G. (1994, March). PsychoanalyticBased Psychotherapy I. Carpinteria, CA: Pacifica Graduate Institute.

Linker, G. (1994). The function of imagery in psychotherapy. (Paper submitted for publication.)

Loewald, H.W. (2000). *The Essential Loewald: Collected Papers and Monographs.* Hagerstown, MD: University Publishing Group.

Lorenzer, A. and Orban, P. (1995). Transitional objects and phenomena: Socialization and symbolization. In S.A. Grolnick and L. Barkin (eds.), *Between Reality and Fantasy: Winnicott's Concepts of Transitional Objects and Phenomena* (pp. 469–483). Northvale, NJ: Jason Aronson.

Lowinski, N.R. (1992). Stories *from the Motherline: Reclaiming the Mother-daughter Bond, Finding Our Feminine Souls*. Los Angeles: Jeremy P. Tarcher.

Mahler, M. (1994). On sadness and grief in infancy and childhood. In *Infantile Psychosis & Early Contributions: The Selected Papers of Margaret S. Mahler* (Vol. 1) (pp. 261–279). Northvale, NJ: Jason Aronson, Inc.

Mayer, E.L. (2008). *Extraordinary Knowing: Science, Skepticism and the Inexplicable Powers of the Human Mind.* New York: Bantam Books.

Miller, J.B. (1991). The development of women's sense of self. In J.V. Jordan et al., *Women's Growth in Connection.* New York: Guilford Press.

Modell, A. (1996). The synergy of memory, affects and metaphor. *Journal of Analytical Psychology*, 42: 105–119.

Mogenson, G. (1992). *Greeting the Angels: An Imaginal View of the Mourning Process.* Amityville, New York: Baywood Publishing Company, Inc.

Murray, G. (1955). *Five Stages of Greek Religion.* Garden City, NY: Doubleday.

Nagy, G. (1990). *Greek Mythology and Poetics.* Ithaca, NY: Cornell University Press.

Neumann, E. (1973). *The Origins and History of Consciousness* (3rd ed.). Princeton, NJ: Princeton University Press.

Nilsson, M. (1940). *Greek Popular Religion.* New York: Columbia University Press.

Ogden, T.H. (1989). *The Primitive Edge of Experience.* Northvale, NJ: Jason Aronson.

Ogden, T.H. (1993). *The Matrix of the Mind: Object Relations and the Psychoanalytic Dialogue.* Northvale, NJ: Jason Aronson.

Ogden, T.H. (2001). *Conversations at the Frontier of Dreaming* (pp. 203–236). Northvale, NJ: Jason Aronson.

Onians, R.B. (1951). *The Origins of European Thought* (2nd ed.). Cambridge, UK: Cambridge University Press.

Ornstein, P.H. (1980). Self-psychology and the concept of health. In A. Goldberg (ed.), *Advances in Self Psychology.* New York: International Universities Press.

Ovid (1958). *The Metamorphoses*. (H. Gregory, trans.). New York: Viking Press.

Padel, R. (1992). *In and Out of the Greek Mind: Greek Images of the Tragic Self.* Princeton, NJ: Princeton University Press.

Padel, R. (1995). *Whom Gods Destroy: Elements of Greek and Tragic Madness*. Princeton, NJ: Princeton University Press.

Panajian, A. (1994, Winter). "Clinical Practicum I." Carpinteria, CA: Pacifica Graduate Institute.

Parke, H.W. and Wormell, D.E.W. (1956). *The Delphic Oracle* (Vols. 1–2). Oxford: Oxford University Press.

Perera, S.B. (1981). *Descent to the Goddess: A Way of Initiation for Women.* Toronto, Canada: Inner City Books.

Philips, A. (1994). On flirtation, in *Futures* (p. 156). Cambridge, MA: Harvard University Press.

Plato (1961). The Republic (P. Shorey, trans.) In E. Hamilton and H. Cairns (eds.), *The Collected Dialogues of Plato.* New York: Pantheon Books.

Richardson, N.J. (ed.) (1974). *The Homeric Hymn to Demeter.* Oxford: Oxford University Press.

Riker, J.H. (1997). *Ethics and the Discovery of the Unconscious*. Albany, NY: State University of New York Press.

Romanyshyn, R. (1992). *Technology as Symptom and Dream.* Routledge: London.

Romanyshyn, R. (October, 1995). Unpublished Lecture. Carpinteria, CA: Pacifica Graduate Institute.

Romanyshyn, R. (December, 1995). Unpublished Lecture. Carpinteria, CA: Pacifica Graduate Institute.

Romilly, J. (1975). *Magic and Rhetoric in Ancient Greece.* Cambridge, MA: Harvard University Press.

Schwartz-Salant, N. (1988). Archetypal foundations of projective identification. *Journal of Analytical Psychology*, 33: 39–64.

Schwartz-Salant, N. (1989). *The Borderline Personality: Vision and Healing*. Wihnette, IL: Chiron Publications.

Schwartz-Salant, N. and Stein, M. (eds.) (1991). *Liminality and Transitional Phenomena.* The Chiron Clinical Series. Wilmette, II: Chiron Press.

Sculley, V.T. (1962). *The Earth, the Temple and the Gods*. New Haven, CT: Yale University Press.

Seaford, R. (1995). *Reciprocity and Ritual: Homer and Tragedy in the Developing City-state*. New York: Oxford University Press.

Segal, C. (1981). *Tragedy and Civilization: An Interpretation of Sophocles*. Cambridge, MA: Harvard University Press.

Segal, C. (1982). *Dionysiac Poetics and Euripides' Bacchae*. Princeton: Princeton University Press.

Segal, C. (1986). *Interpreting Greek Tragedy: Myth, Poetry, Text*. Ithaca, NY: Cornell University Press.

Segal, H. (1964). *Introduction to the World of Melanie Klein*. New York: Basic Books.

Simon, B. (1978). *Mind and Madness in Ancient Greece*. Ithaca, NY: Cornell University Press.

Slater, P.E. (1968). *The Glory of Hera: Greek Mythology and the Greek Family*. Boston, MA: Beacon Press.

Snell, B. (1960). *The Discovery of the Mind* (T.G. Rosenmeyer, trans.). Oxford: Oxford University Press. (Original work published 1953.)

Sophocles (1973). *Sophocles I: Oedipus the King* (D. Grene, trans.) *Oedipus at Colonus* (R. Fitzgerald, trans.), *Antigone* (E. Wyckoff, trans.), Chicago, IL: University of Chicago.

Sophoclis Fabulae (1975). (A.C. Pearson, ed.). Ely House, London: Oxford University Press.

Stanford, W.B. (1983). *Greek Tragedy and the Emotions*. London: Routledge & Kegan Paul.

Stern, D.N. (1985). *The Interpersonal World of the Infant: A View from Psychoanalysis and Developmental Psychology*. New York: Basic Books.

Stolorow, R.D. (2007). *Trauma and Human Existence: Autobiographical, Psychoanalytic, and Philosophical Reflections*. New York, London: Analytic Press.

Stolorow, R.D., Brandchaft, B., and Atwood, G.E. (1987). *Psychoanalytic Treatment: An Intersubjective Approach*. Hillsdale, NJ: Analytic Press.

Stolorow, R.D., Atwood, G.E., and Brandchaft, B. (eds.) (1994). *The Intersubjective Perspective*. Northvale, NJ: Jason Aronson, Inc.

Stolz, B.A. and R.S. Shannon (eds.) (1976). *Oral Literature and the Formula*. Ann Arbor, MI: University of Michigan Press.

Sullivan, H.S. (1940). *Conceptions of Modem Psychiatry*. New York: Norton.

Surrey, J.L., Kaplan, A.G., and Jordan, J.V. (1990). *Empathy Revisited* (Work in Progress #40). Wellesley, MA: The Stone Center, Wellesley College.

Tolpin, M. (1971). On the beginnings of a cohesive self: An application of the concept of transmuting internalization to the study of the transitional object and signal anxiety. *Psychoanalytic Study of the Child*, 26: 316–352.

Thucydides (1951). *The Peloponnesian War* (J.H. Finley, Jr., ed.). New York: Modern Library.

Vernant, J.P. (1983a). Personal identity and religion. In *Myth and Thought Among the Greeks* (pp. 321–341). London: Routledge & Kegan Paul.

Vernant, J.P. (1983b). The psychological category of the double. In *Myth and Thought Among the Greeks* (pp. 303–321). London: Routledge & Kegan Paul.

Vemant, J.P. (1991a). The birth of images. In F.I. Zeitlin (ed.), *Mortals and Immortals* (pp. 164–185). Princeton: Princeton University Press.

Vernant, J.P. (1991b). From the "presentification" of the invisible to the imitation of appearance. In F.I. Zeitlin (ed.), *Mortals and Immortals: Collected Essays* (pp. 151–163). Princeton, NJ: Princeton University Press.

Vernant, J.P. (1991c). Mortals and immortals: The body of the divine. In F.I. Zeitlin (ed.), *Mortals and Immortals: Collected Essays* (pp. 27–49). Princeton, NJ: Princeton University Press.

Vemant, J.P. (1991d). Psuche: Simulacrum of the body or image of the divine? In F.I. Zeitlin (ed.), *Mortals and Immortals: Collected Essays* (pp. 186–194). Princeton, NJ: Princeton University Press.

Vernant, J.P. and Vidal-Naquet, P. (1988). Intimations of the will in Greek tragedy. In *Myth and Tragedy in Ancient Greece* (pp. 49–84). New York: Urzone, Inc.

Wheelwright, P. (ed.) (1966). *The Presocratics.* New York: Odyssey Press.

Winnicott, D.W. (1958a). Aggression in relation to emotional development. In *Through Paediatrics to Psycho-analysis* (pp. 204–218). New York: Basic Books.

Winnicott, D.W. (1958b). Primary maternal preoccupation. In *Through Paediatrics to Psycho-analysis* (pp. 300–306). New York: Basic Books.

Winnicott, D.W. (1958c). The manic defense. In *Through Paediatrics to Psycho-analysis* (pp. 129–145). New York: Basic Books.

Winnicott, D.W. (1958d). Transitional objects and transitional phenomena. In *Through Paediatrics to Psycho-analysis* (pp. 229–243). New York: Basic Books.

Winnicott, D.W. (1965a). The capacity for concern. In *The Maturational Processes and the Facilitating Environment: Studies in the Theory of Emotional Development* (pp. 73–81). New York: International Universities Press.

Winnicott, D.W. (1965b). Ego distortion in terms of true and false self. In *The Maturational Processes and the Facilitating Environment: Studies in the Theory of Emotional Development* (pp. 140–153). New York: International Universities Press.

Winnicott, D.W. (1971). Dreaming, fantasying and living. In *Playing and Reality* (pp. 26–38). London: Routledge.

Winnicott, D.W. (1971). Transitional objects and transitional phenomena. In *Playing and Reality* (pp. 1–25). London: Routledge.

Winnicott, D.W. (1971). The use of an object and relating through identifications. In *Playing and Reality* (pp. 86–94). London: Routledge.

Wolf, E.S. (1988). *Treating the Self: Elements of Clinical Self Psychology.* New York: Guilford Press.

Wolkstein, D. and Kramer, S.N. (1983). *Inanna: Queen of Heaven and Earth: Her Stories and Hymns from Sumer.* New York: Harper & Row.

Zabriskie, B. (1997). Thawing the "frozen accidents": The archetypal view in countertransference. *Journal of Analytical Psychology*, 42: 25–40.

Zuntz, G. (1971). *Persephone: Three Essays on Religion and Thought in Magna Graecia.* Oxford: Oxford University Press.

Index

For Product Safety Concerns and Information please contact our EU
representative GPSR@taylorandfrancis.com
Taylor & Francis Verlag GmbH, Kaufingerstraße 24, 80331 München, Germany

www.ingramcontent.com/pod-product-compliance
Ingram Content Group UK Ltd.
Pitfield, Milton Keynes, MK11 3LW, UK
UKHW022316250926
475702UK00046B/891
* 9 7 8 1 0 3 2 3 7 5 5 1 9 *